SMART INFUSION PUMPS

Implementation, Management, and Drug Libraries

Pamela K. Phelps, Pharm.D., FASHP
Director, Clinical Pharmacy Services
Fairview Health Services
Adjunct Associate Professor,
    University of Minnesota College of Pharmacy
Minneapolis, Minnesota

American Society of Health-System Pharmacists®
Bethesda, Maryland

Any correspondence regarding this publication should be sent to the publisher, American Society of Health-System Pharmacists, 7272 Wisconsin Avenue, Bethesda, MD 20814, attention: Special Publishing.

The information presented herein reflects the opinions of the contributors and advisors. It should not be interpreted as an official policy of ASHP or as an endorsement of any product.

Because of ongoing research and improvements in technology, the information and its applications contained in this text are constantly evolving and are subject to the professional judgment and interpretation of the practitioner due to the uniqueness of a clinical situation. The editors, contributors, and ASHP have made reasonable efforts to ensure the accuracy and appropriateness of the information presented in this document. However, any user of this information is advised that the editors, contributors, advisors, and ASHP are not responsible for the continued currency of the information, for any errors or omissions, and/or for any consequences arising from the use of the information in the document in any and all practice settings. Any reader of this document is cautioned that ASHP makes no representation, guarantee, or warranty, express or implied, as to the accuracy and appropriateness of the information contained in this document and specifically disclaims any liability to any party for the accuracy and/or completeness of the material or for any damages arising out of the use or non-use of any of the information contained in this document.

Director, Special Publishing: Jack Bruggeman

Senior Editorial Project Manager: Dana A. Battaglia

Editorial Resources Manager: Bill Fogle

Cover Design: David Wade

Composition: Carol A. Barrer

Library of Congress Cataloging-in-Publication Data

Smart infusion pumps : implementation, management, and drug libraries / [edited by] Pamela K. Phelps, PharmD.

   p. ; cm.

Includes bibliographical references and index.

ISBN 978-1-58528-230-2

1. Drug infusion pumps. I. Phelps, Pamela K., editor. II. American Society of Health-System Pharmacists, issuing body.

[DNLM: 1. Infusion Pumps. 2. Pharmaceutical Preparations--administration & dosage. WB 354]

RM170.5.S63 2011

615'.19--dc22

2010046987

ISBN 978-1-58528-230-2

Dedication

For Ben, without whom my work is impossible.

Preface

On April 23, 2010, the FDA launched its "Initiative to Reduce Infusion Pump Risks." This initiative, in response to a plethora of pump defects and recalls, aims to establish additional premarket requirements for external infusion pumps. Defects have been identified with hardware (mechanical, electrical), software, and with the user interfaces. Shortly after this FDA initiative was announced, my editor at ASHP called me and asked the question, "Is this the right time to release a book on smart pumps?" My answer was "Yes, the need remains the same for those who must evaluate, implement, and manage smart infusion pumps." I sincerely hope that this book provides timely advice and benefit to those who use it.

With this book, the authors and I take you through our journey in the purchase and implementation of smart pumps. Chapter 1 addresses the need for smart pumps. While the need may seem obvious to pharmacists and nurses, helpful references are provided to help you "state your case" to obtain the necessary resources to purchase and implement new infusion pumps. Chapter 2 describes the process that our health system went through to make a smart pump choice. This includes the request for proposal, pump attribute evaluation, and value analysis. An example of a request for proposal and pump "scoring list" is provided. Chapter 3 describes the use of human factors techniques such as usability testing and failure mode and effects analysis to aid in the decision-making process. Using these techniques will also help you to identify any failure modes with your chosen pump. Identifying these failure modes prior to implementation is crucial to development of meaningful training materials and safe and effective processes. In Chapter 4, suggested guiding principles are offered. Some of these developed over time, when we were in the process of decision-making and said "we should really articulate our philosophy on that point." These are things that we said later "we wish we knew that from the start." Establishing guiding principles from the start will benefit the health system immensely. Chapter 5 represents our general pump library with associated high and low limits. Not all pumps will require low limits. This library is offered as a starting point. We expect that health systems will learn more about their practices over time, and the pump library will evolve. In addition, new drug releases and new literature will create the need for pump library changes. Chapter 6 outlines the unique issues encountered with patient controlled analgesia (PCA). Background information and literature are provided to support the PCA pump library recommendations. Chapter 7 deals specifically with the pediatric drug library. A dedicated pediatric library is required due to higher risk, weight-based dosing, different infusion concentrations, smaller volumes, and different types of pumps. Chapter 8 deals with the considerations in setting up separate care areas within the pump library. Issues of standardized versus non-standardized drug libraries are addressed. This is where pump library medication and library number limitations will impact on decision-making. Information Services capacity will also come into play, when deciding on care areas. Chapter 9 offers advice on preparation and education for go-live. Strategies for gaining buy-in, training and encouragement are given. Preparation, education, and communication are some of the most important aspects of pump implementation. Chapter 10 deals exclusively with the impact that pump changes will have on the pharmacy sterile products or compounding areas. Considerations in these areas include any process changes, standardization of infusion concentrations, sterile compounding, storage, label printing, bar coding, and assuring product quality. Chapter 11 addresses the process for pump updates. With newer pump technology, frequent updates of the pump library become a part of your regular processes. Steps in these processes will need to be articulated to the supply chain staff, biomedical services, information services staff, and nursing and pharmacy staffs. Since the electronic medical record, medication administration record, flow sheets and order sets are so interrelated, these processes can be quite complex. They therefore deserve a great deal of thought and inter-departmental communication. Chapter 12 deals with maintaining the quality of pump utilization after the implementation. Report writing and analysis will need to be done to ensure compliance with the pump library. Reports can also tell you the quality of your pump library, and what "tweaks" will need to be made to ensure compliance. Reports can also tell you about "good catches" that have been made and errors avoided. Circle this information back to senior leaders to validate the pump investment. Circle it back to the front-line staff to show how the pump benefits the end users. Finally, Chapter 13 offers a process for decision-making for pump updates. Flow diagrams for decision steps are included. As stated earlier, this process involves many disciplines and departments. With so many "moving parts," we developed checklists for each department to make sure we are following our most efficient and safe processes. This activity will bring your hospital's inter-departmental sense of teamwork to a new level, which can be quite rewarding.

The journey continues. Pump technology will continue to evolve, as new features become available, and as the FDA rolls out the new initiative for furthering pump safety. Be prepared to continue to learn and make changes as this happens. I wish you the best of luck on your own journey.

Pamela Phelps
2010

Foreword

Over the past 10 years, there has been an explosion of advances in the medical device industry. Needed technologies have been developed that have changed the practice of pharmacy and made it safer for medications to be distributed and administered. The improvement of intravenous (IV) pump technology is a great example of how these devices have matured over the past decade. Going from a device that calculated the infusion rate by counting the number of drops per minute to one that will calculate the infusion rate on the pump and send usage data wirelessly is remarkable. There have been changes, and I expect the next decade to hold even more promise as these pumps become more user-friendly with the potential for reducing medication errors.

I first got involved in this area when I was asked in 2003 to conduct a beta test of one of the smart pumps. We studied it over 14 days in our intensive care units. While the evaluation of this technology on the patients and healthcare workers was one aspect of the study, the preparation to get ready for this was even more difficult. Our organization needed to be educated on the value of this technology (which meant informing leaders of the potential dangers with the current system), creating standard concentrations and dosing parameters for a drug library, and getting these infusion recommendations approved by the P&T committee.

When we embarked on this study, many of the current smart pumps were not on the market. In addition, there were no printed resources to assist with the development of the drug libraries. Having access to chapters like those contained within this book would have been helpful to our organization and saved a tremendous amount of time!

Many organizations still have not implemented smart pumps and this book will be a great resource to them. Each hospital in this situation should read this book in advance to prepare for the implementation of smart pumps. The chapter authors are well-respected practitioners and covered the breadth of issues within their respective chapters. Even if your organization has adopted smart pumps, there might be some delivery modalities (pediatric infusions, patient controlled analgesia, or epidurals) where smart pump technology has not been implemented yet. This book would be a valuable asset for these different populations. Finally, there are many pearls included in each chapter to help organizations that have fully embraced smart pumps find ways to improve utilization of the dosing libraries and reduce medication errors in their respective organizations.

The book is presented in an easy to read format with very practical and useful information contained in each chapter. The first chapter has an example of a return on investment calculation that can be easily utilized to upgrade to smart pump technology. The second chapter has a valuable sample request for proposal and listing of desirable features of infusion pumps. This information is required for any review of IV pumps and many times difficult and time consuming to develop internally. Having detailed examples makes this book that much more worthwhile to organizations.

Another useful tool is the practice tips found at the end of each chapter. These statements are concise, practical, and applicable to all types of organizations. Further, the philosophical tenets embedded throughout Chapter 4 regarding implementation strategies will force any reader to contemplate whether their organization has maximized the full benefit of smart pumps. Finally, including chapters solely focused on patient controlled analgesia, pediatrics, and compounding gives a breadth to the applicability of this book to all practice sites.

While the past decade has seen a tremendous amount of development in smart pump technology, the next decade holds even more promise. With regulatory changes coming to the device approval process, the opportunity for smart pumps to become fully integrated into the electronic health record, the potential to interface with IV room workload technology and have seamless delivery of medications, and the further development into areas where this technology is still immature (i.e., chemotherapy delivery), there is great promise in the next decade. This is a fantastic opportunity for the profession of pharmacy to take a leadership role in smart pump technology and this book serves as a critical resource to do that.

Congratulations to Pam Phelps for leading the initiative that developed this needed resource and for identifying the authors who wrote excellent chapters. Having most of the authors coming from one practice arena, the University of Minnesota Medical Center and Fairview Health Services, provides optimism that one organization can fully implement these strategies. This book can be an aid for organizations maximizing their use of smart pump technology. By following the recommendations contained within, patient care at your institution will be improved and medication errors will be reduced.

This is exactly what we found when we conducted the beta test years ago. Our organization saw the dramatic results from the drug library limits and we became early adopters of this technology. I recommend this book to anyone looking to improve medication delivery in their organizations and minimize medication errors. Even if you feel like you have fully adopted these devices, there might be some ideas not considered that can further improve the use in your hospital. I know I found that to be true.

Stephen F. Eckel, Pharm.D., MHA, BCPS, FAPhA, FASHP
Assistant Director of Pharmacy
University of North Carolina Hospitals
Clinical Assistant Professor
University of North Carolina Eshelman School of Pharmacy

Table of Contents

Contributors

John R. Bloomfield, Ph.D.
University of Minnesota
Minneapolis, Minnesota

Michelle L. Borchart, Pharm.D.
Clinical Pharmacist
University of Minnesota Medical Center
Minneapolis, Minnesota

Burnis D. Breland, M.S., Pharm.D., FASHP
Director of Pharmacy and Clinical Research
Columbus Regional Healthcare System

Adjunct Professor of Pharmacy Practice
Auburn University Harrison School of Pharmacy
The Medical Center, Inc.
Columbus, Georgia

Carolyn K. Carlson, Pharm.D.
Clinical Pharmacist
University of Minnesota Medical Center
Minneapolis, Minnesota

Melissa Carlson, Pharm.D., BCPS
Pharmacy Pediatric Team Leader
University of Minnesota Medical Center
Minneapolis, Minnesota

Craig E. Else, Pharm.D.
Pharmacy Director
Fairview Ridges Hospital
Burnsville, Minnesota

Virginia L. Ghafoor, Pharm.D.
Clinical Pharmacist, Pain Management
University of Minnesota Medical Center
Minneapolis, Minnesota

Kathleen A. Harder, Senior Research Associate
College of Design
Minneapolis, Minnesota

Gregg F. Herrmann, R.Ph.

Manager, Pharmacy Informatics
Fairview Pharmacy Services
Minneapolis, Minnesota

Patty L. Kleinke, R.N., BAN

Supply Chain
Fairview Health Services
Supply Chain Administration
Minneapolis, Minnesota

Susan M. Kleppin, R.Ph.

Pharmacy Manager
Waukesha Memorial Hospital
Waukesha Wisconsin

Carol S. Manchester, MSN, ACNS, BC-ADM, CDE

Diabetes Clinical Nurse Specialist
University of Minnesota Medical Center, Fairview
Minneapolis, Minnesota

University of Minnesota Amplatz Children's Hospital, Fairview
Minneapolis, Minnesota

Pamela K. Phelps, Pharm.D., FASHP

Director, Clinical Pharmacy Services
Fairview Health Services

Adjunct Associate Professor, University of Minnesota College of Pharmacy
Minneapolis, Minnesota

Janell M. Schultz, Pharm.D.

Pharmacy Manager
St. Francis Regional Medical Center
Shakopee, Minnesota

Angela Skoglund, Pharm.D., BCPS

Clinical Pharmacist—Pediatrics
Clinical Assistant Professor, University of Minnesota College of Pharmacy
Minneapolis, Minnesota

Reviewers

Tammy Cohen, Pharm.D

Director of Pharmacy, Baylor Heart and Vascular Hospital
Dallas, Texas

Cris Denniston, Pharm.D

Director of Pharmacy, Cortland Regional Medical Center
Cortland, New York

Stephen F. Eckel, Pharm.D, MHA, BCPS, FAPhA, FASHP

Assistant Director of Pharmacy, Residency Program Director
University of North Carolina Hospitals

and

Clinical Assistant Professor, Eshelman School of Pharmacy
University of North Carolina at Chapel Hill
Chapel Hill, North Carolina

John C. Mattern, Pharm.D

Pharmacy Manager, Stoughton Hospital
Stoughton, Wisconsin

Kelly A. Michienzi, Pharm.D

Clinical Pharmacy Coordinator, Women & Children's Hospital of Buffalo
Buffalo, New York

Justification for Smart Pump Technology

Pamela K. Phelps

Key Terms

Infusion pump—device that uses pressure to deliver specific volumes of fluid; used for fluid, blood, and medication administration.

Smart infusion pumps—a new generation of infusion pumps that incorporates dose limiting software into the pump hardware; this software is designed to prevent infusion-related programming errors. The Joint Commission, in the 2006 National Patient Safety Goals, defined a smart pump as a "parenteral infusion pump equipped with IV medication error-prevention software that alerts operators or interrupts the infusion process when a pump setting is programmed outside of pre-configured limits." Smart pumps are designed to recognize prescription errors, dose misinterpretations, and keypad programming error.

Dose error reduction system (DERS)—term used to describe software built into intelligent infusion devices that is designed to catch dosing or administration errors. The software alerts the user if pre-determined high dosage limits are exceeded, or if entry is below pre-determined low dosage limits.

Return on investment (ROI)—performance measure used to evaluate the efficiency of an investment.

MAUDE—the Manufacturer and User Facility Device Experience is an online database maintained by the FDA. MAUDE data represents voluntary reports of adverse events involving medical devices.

510(k) clearance—Section 510(k) of the Food, Drug, and Cosmetic Act requires device manufacturers to notify the FDA of their intent to market a medical device at least 90 days in advance. High-risk devices are designated at Class III, and require 510(k) clearance prior to marketing.

The Need for New Technology

Purchasing and implementing intelligent infusion devices ("smart pumps") may seem at first to be a daunting and expensive task. But examining the data on infusion related errors brings us to a rapid conclusion that it is a worthwhile endeavor. Consider the Institute of Medicine Report "To Err is Human," issued in 1999.[1] This oft-quoted report stated that 44,000 to 98,000 error-related deaths occurred per year in the hospital environment. As many as 70% of these errors are preventable.[2] Medication errors comprise the highest percentage of non-surgical errors and are consistently reported to be approximately 19%.[2-4] One author estimated that medication-related errors are as high as 44% of non-surgical errors.[5] Researchers conducting an AHRQ-funded study at Brigham and Women's Hospital and Massachusetts General Hospital found that, on average, ADEs increased the length of stay by as much as 4.6 days and increased costs up to $4,685.[6]

The most serious medication errors are caused by IV administration of medications.[7] The United States Pharmacopeia operates a national database for reporting medication errors called MedMarx. Data from MedMarx indicates that medication errors involving parenteral medications are three times as likely to cause harm or death when compared to other medication errors.[7] The vast majority (79%) of these errors involving parenteral medications were associated with the intravenous route of administration and occurred at the point of care delivery, during administration of the medication. A systems analysis of adverse drug events performed by Leape et al, revealed proximal causes and systems failures associated with adverse drug events.[8] **Infusion pump** and parenteral delivery problems were identified as a proximal cause in 5% of adverse drug events. All occurred during the nurse administration phase of the drug delivery system. Further, "device use" accounted for 4% of systems failures identified. The most common reason for the administration of a wrong dose of an intravenous medication is an error in programming an IV infusion pump.[9]

Pediatric patients are at an even higher risk of medication errors. Raju[10] examined medication errors in a pediatric intensive care unit and found that medication errors occurred at a rate of 1 for each 6.8 admissions. The frequency of injury from a medication-related error in a pediatric intensive care unit is 3.19%. 60% of these errors were attributed to a nurse error during medication administration.

In healthcare, we traditionally rely upon bedside caregivers for the "Five Rights": administering the right drug to the right patient in the right dose by the right route at the right time. This process is fraught with human error, and may be an unrealistic expectation. Bedside bar-coding, along with intelligent infusion devices will begin the process of eliminating the blame associated with the Five Rights as a cause for medication error and injury. Additionally, the Center for Medicare and Medicaid Services (CMS) is implementing a new initiative, whereby hospitals will no longer be reimbursed for "hospital-acquired" conditions such as pressure ulcers, hospital acquired infections, and certain complications. Private payers will likely follow suit. The Joint Commission White Paper, "Hospital of the Future,"[11] establishes principles to guide technology adoption. Relevant to his discussion are the principles to "use digital technology to support patient-centered hospital care" and "adopt technologies that are labor-saving and integrative across the hospital."

The Institute for Safe Medication Practices[12] advocates the use of health care technology, such as "smart pumps." One of the potentially dangerous practices identified by ISMP is harmful mix-ups among various dosing methods for the drugs in the pump's library. For example, a medication may be infused based on mcg/kg/min on one hospital unit, and infused using mcg/min on another unit. The use of smart pump technology can customize the dose expression according to the specific unit or patient population. Other safety features include unchangeable dosing units once a drug is selected, weight limits, and clinical advisories.[13] ISMP has also identified pump errors based on "double-bumping" keypads and bypassing safety software. "Key Bounce" is listed as a potential cause of pump error in the MAUDE.

What Makes Smart Pumps Smart?

DERS

New pump technology can be contrasted to older pumps by describing the dose error reduction systems (DERS) employed. Typically, the pump software resides on a website, where changes in dose limits can be made. Limits in the pump software will alert the user if drug dose, dosing unit, or dosing rate are outside of usual limits. Dose limits can be "soft" or "hard," and "low" or "high." Note that not all pumps have low limits built into their software, but all vendors have high limits. A "low-soft" limit will alert the user when the dose programmed into the pump is considered lower than is typical. A "low-hard" limit will alert the user when the dose programmed into the pump is considered lower than any recommended dose. A "high-soft" limit will alert the user when the dose programmed into the pump is considered higher than is typical. A "high-hard" limit will alert the user when the dose programmed into the pump is higher than what is allowed by the institution. It is important to consider that "soft" limits can be overridden, and the programmer can proceed with the infusion. While not true for all vendors, some pumps allow overriding "hard" limits with a passcode. In general, a hard limit should force the user to re-program the pump. If the institution chooses a pump with hard limit overriding, this will allow overriding "hard" limits for exceptional situations, such as emergencies. This type of technology is most useful for preventing overt programming errors (for example, a ten-time overdose) or soft-key "double-bumping." Newer pumps have a much greater memory capacity for medication dose programming.

Wireless Technology

Another benefit of the new technology is the ability to update the pump firmware or software using wireless technology. Wireless technology allows for two-way wireless transfer of information. Drug libraries and software updates from the server can be sent by wireless technology to each pump in the institution. Conversely, pump events and alarm logs are sent from the pumps to the server. The wireless technology will allow pump upgrades and drug library changes without having to collect and quarantine pumps. If a pump is in a non-wireless area of the institution, it simply needs to be moved to a wireless area, in order to receive updates.

Data Logs

Finally, the wireless technology records all dose limit events and the clinician response. This allows creation of reports that can be analyzed for error "saves," as well as any nuisance alerts that are being overridden. Most vendors will supply log-analysis software with the product, that allows for "canned" reports to be run on a regular basis. With this information, the pump library can be changed to ensure safety limits, without alerting the caregiver with unnecessary alerts and causing fatigue.

Return on Investment

The need for the new technology is justified based on the patient safety data outlined above. But, smart pumps will also need to be justified financially. This can be accomplished through the use of a **return on investment** (ROI) analysis.[14] An ROI is used to measure the efficiency and profitability of an investment, especially when the "return" may not be realized immediately. A typical ROI displays anticipated gains and losses over a period of 5 years. The equation used for an ROI is listed below:

$$ROI = \frac{\text{gains from investment} - \text{cost of investment}}{\text{cost of investment}}$$

This is usually expressed as a percentage. A percentage or ratio greater than zero indicates that the returns are greater than the costs, and therefore justifies the expenditure. A basic example of an ROI template for smart pumps is demonstrated in Figure 1-1.

Once pumps are implemented, data collected from pump data logs may indicate additional savings in drug utilization.[14] Follow-up documentation should demonstrate the actual reduction in intravenous adverse drug events, circling back to the return on investment.

	Year 1	Year 2	Year 3	Year 4	Year 5	Total
Pump purchase or rental	($500,000)	($10,000)	($10,000)	($10,000)	($10,000)	($540,000)
Additional staff for implementation and maintenance (salary)	($50,000)	0	0	0	0	($50,000)
Savings on disposable (syringes, tubing, etc.)	$20,000	$20,600	$21,218	$21,854	$22,510	$106,182
Savings on IV solutions	$20,000	$20,600	$21,218	$21,854	$22,510	$106,182
Number of avoided ADEs	25	25	25	25	25	
Cost per ADE	$9992*	$10,591	$11,608	$12,304	$13,043	
Cost avoidance, all ADEs	$249,800	$264,775	$290,200	$307,600	$326,075	$1,438,450
Return on investment						$1.79 or 179%

*Cost savings identified in reference 6, inflated 6% per year to year 2010.

Assumptions with this model:

Capital outlay is largest in Year 1. Year 2–5 investments are for additional pumps that may be needed for growth.

The additional staff budget is incremental to current staff only. For example, you may need a project manager for implementation in the first year. After the first year, staff who are currently handling pump maintenance will continue to do so.

A new pump contract will yield savings with disposables and with IV solutions.

The hospital in this example has documented 25 serious adverse drug events per year that will be avoided with smart pump.

Figure 1-1. Example of an ROI (return on investment) template.

Pump Attributes

Attributes of smart pumps should be compared between various brands of pumps. The technology changes quickly, necessitating frequent updates of pump specifications. Examples of attributes that should be evaluated include wireless features, single-channel versus double-channel, number of libraries and medications per library, bolus limits, visibility of alerts, availability of a syringe connection, screen readability, infusion rate limits, dose limits for a secondary infusion and report writing. Pharmacy and supply chain should also evaluate the vendor attributes to ensure that all infusion needs can be met. These attributes include proprietary tubing, bag-based drug delivery systems, small- and large-volume infusion fluids, and parenteral nutrition supplies and compounders.

Challenges in the Marketplace

Numerous reports to the FDA through the MAUDE, including significant recalls, has caused healthcare providers to re-evaluate their pump utilization. There were 132 product recalls for large volume pumps between 2003 and 2008. Recalls included many types of failures, including power cord failure, inaccurate flow rates, occlusion warnings, and blank screen errors. Healthcare providers involved in the purchase or maintenance of IV pump technology should become familiar with the MAUDE database and the FDA website. Whenever significant upgrades to the pump technology take place (particularly when the upgrade is a "fix" for a pump malfunction), these upgrades should obtain 510(k) clearance from the FDA.

On April 23, 2010, FDA launched its "Initiative to Reduce Infusion Pump Risks."[15] The initiative, in response to a plethora of pump defects and recalls, aims to establish addition pre-market requirements for external infusion pumps. Defects have been identified with hardware (mechanical, electrical), software, and user interfaces. From 2005 through 2009, FDA received 56,000 reports of adverse events associated with infusion pump use. FDA estimates that more than 500 deaths are attributable to pump defects.[16] In addition to establishing stricter requirements for pump approval, FDA will offer to test software during pre-market review and increase user awareness of strategies to mitigate risk with existing pumps. FDA has also drafted a guidance document for pre-market notification submissions entitled "Total Product Life Cycle: Infusion Pump."[17] The guidance document advises the pump industry to conduct extensive pre-marketing testing using simulation and human factors analysis, and to devise risk mitigation strategies. Then, on April 30, 2010, FDA sent a letter to Baxter ordering the company to recall and destroy their Colleague® Volumetric Infusion Pumps used in the United States.

Clearly, these facts represent challenges in the marketplace. Pump manufacturers will be challenged to provide more proof of safety and testing for their products, which may mean a slower progression of new products to the market. Manufacturers will have to move swiftly to ensure that an adequate supply of usable pumps are available to meet patient care needs.

Conclusion

There is compelling evidence that new safety systems are needed for IV administration of medications. A drug error reduction system is a desirable part of any new intelligent infusion device. While this system cannot prevent all errors, it is a major step forward in the development of fail-safe systems for drug administration at the bedside. Despite current marketplace challenges, the healthcare system and public will continue to demand fail-safe smart pumps in order to meet patient care needs. Photographs of commonly used smart pumps are in Figure 1-2.

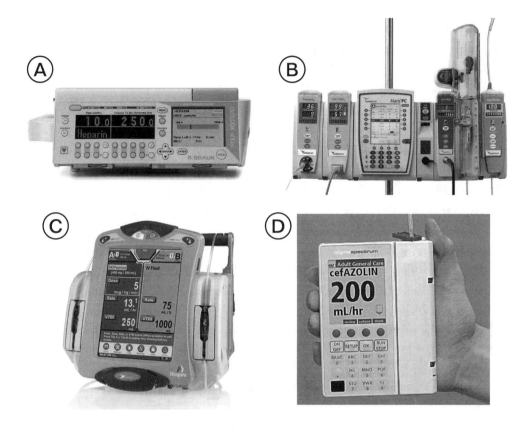

Figure 1-2. Examples of common types of smart infusion pumps. *Source:* (A) Printed with permission of B. Braun Medical, Inc. (B) Printed with permission of Cardinal Health, Inc. (C) Printed with permission of Hospira, Inc. (D) Printed with permission of Baxter International, Inc.

On-Line Resources for Vendor Evaluation

KLAS Enterprises, LLC, provides technology vendor performance reviews, including smart pumps. This resource is available online, by subscription. ECRI Institute provides product evaluations online (membership may be required for access).

Practice Tips

- Gain administrative buy-in for the implementation of smart pump technology. Use current literature as well as institution-specific "stories" of how pump errors have contributed to sub-optimal care in the institution.
- Validate economic benefit with an ROI analysis.
- Link with Information Services to validate wireless capabilities.
- Identify nursing leadership champions to support implementation of smart pumps.

References

1. Kohn LT, Corrigan JM, Donaldson MS. To err is human: building a safer health system. A report of the Committee on Quality of Health Care in America. Washington, DC: National Academy Press; 2000.

2. Leape LL, Lawthers AG, Brennan, et al. Preventing Medical Injury. *Qual Rev Bull.* 1993;19:144-149.

3. Thomas, EJ, Studdert, DM, Burstin, HR, et al. Incidence and types of adverse events and negligent care in Utah and Colorado. *Med Care.* 2000;38(3):261-271.

4. Leape LL, Brennan TA, Laird N, et al. The nature of adverse events in hospitalized patients: results of the Harvard Medical Practice Study II. *N Engl J Med.* 1991;324:377-384.

5. Bedell SE, Deitz DC, Leeman D, et al. Incidence and characteristics of preventable iatrogenic cardiac arrests. *JAMA.* 1991;265:2815-2820.

6. Bates DW, Spell N, Cullen DJ, et al. The costs of adverse drug events in hospitalized patients. *JAMA.* 1997;277(4):307-311.

7. Hicks RW, Becker SC. An overview of intravenous-related medication administration errors as reported to MED-MARX, a national medication error-reporting program. *J Infus Nurs.* 2006;29:20-27.

8. Leape LL, Bates DW, Cullen DJ, et al. Systems analysis of adverse drug events. *JAMA.* 1995;274(1):35-43.

9. Adachi W, Lodolce AE. Use of failure mode and effects analysis in improving the safety of IV drug administration. *AJHP.* 2005;62:917-920.

10. Raju TNK, Kecskes S, Thornton, JP. Medication errors in neonatal and paediatric intensive-care units. *Lancet.* 1989;2(8659):374-376.

11. The Joint Commission. Health Care at the Crossroads: Guiding principles for the development of the hospital of the future. Available at: http://www.jointcommission.org/PublicPolicy/future.htm. Accessed February 25, 2009.

12. Cohen MR, Schneider P, Niemi K. Effective approaches to standardization and implementation of smart pump technology. ISMP Newsletter. 2007.

13. Lack of standard dosing methods contributes to IV errors. ISMP Newsletter. August 22, 2007.

14. Danello SH, Maddox RR, Schaack GJ. Intravenous infusion safety technology: return on investment. *Hosp Pharm.* 2009;44:680.

15. White Paper: Infusion Pump Improvement Initiative. April 2010. Center for Devices and Radiological Health, U.S. Food and Drug Administration. Accessed online June 2, 2010.

16. FDA News Release. FDA Issues Statement on Baxter's Recall of Colleague Infusion Pumps. May 3, 2010. Accessed online June 4, 2010.

17. Guidance for Industry and FDA Staff. Total Product Life Cycle: Infusion Pump: Premarket Notification (510K) Submissions. U.S. Food and Drug Administration. April 23, 2010. Accessed online June 2, 2010.

Choosing a Pump: The Request for Proposal and Value Analysis

Pamela K. Phelps and Patty L. Kleinke

Key Terms

Critical criteria—criteria chosen by a selection team. These criteria, when present, are thought to bring a higher value to the object being evaluated.

MAUDE database—the Manufacturer and User Facility Device Experience is an online database maintained by the FDA. MAUDE data represents voluntary reports of adverse events involving medical devices.

Request for proposal—request for proposal (referred to as RFP) is an invitation for suppliers, often through a bidding process, to submit a proposal for a specific commodity or service.

Value analysis—systematic, objective means to measure the value of an object (usability divided by cost) in comparison to other like objects.

Weighted decision matrix—the process of assigning numerical values to object attributes; the higher the number, the more important the attribute. If an object performs exceptionally well in an attribute with a high matrix value, it is thought to provide more value overall.

The first step in choosing a pump for your health system is choosing a team to develop the critical criteria that must be met by the pump. Team members should include representatives from nursing, pharmacy, anesthesia, biomedical, information services, and supply chain. If applicable, representatives from home infusion and patient safety (or risk management) should participate. Identifying members who are "at the bedside" will benefit the team in pump selection. The goal of the team will be to identify critical criteria for large volume pumps, patient-controlled analgesia pumps, syringe pumps, and epidural pumps. Primary goals are to improve quality and safety, to drive standardization in practice and patient care, and to position the health system for future needs. A structured evaluation process consists of a detailed clinical features matrix, clinician usability testing, and in-depth failure mode and effects analysis (FMEA). Usability testing and FMEA will be discussed in the next chapter.

The second step in the process was to develop a request for proposal, also known as an RFP. An RFP is an invitation for suppliers, often through a bidding process, to submit a proposal for a specific commodity or service (see Figure 2-1).[1] RFPs are sent to known vendors of the product or service and given a due date for delivery of their proposal, or bid. Typically, the institution sending the RFP will be very detailed regarding the information that they want to see from the supplier. The institution sending the RFP will also provide a detailed description of the goods and services they are seeking, the scope of implementation, equipment and personnel requested, and customer service expectations. Additional information requested may be the history and vision of the supplier company, the financial health of the supplier company, technical capabilities of the equipment or personnel, and references from others who have used the company's goods or services. Other sources of information regarding pump attributes can be found through the ECRI Institute and KLAS®. The ECRI Institute is a non-profit organization that conducts evidence-based evaluations of medical procedures, devices, drugs, and processes. The ECRI Institute has been designated an Evidence Based Practice Center by the U.S. Agency for Healthcare Research and Quality (AHRQ). KLAS® is an independently owned and operated company that evaluates and researches healthcare technology performance. These useful on-line resources are available by subscription, and can be extremely helpful.

A sample of an infusion pump RFP is represented in Figure 2-1. A sample of pump criteria is in Table 2-1.

After the RFPs have been completed and returned by suppliers, the team will evaluate the suppliers' goods and services to determine the next steps. The team will need to decide which suppliers meet essential criteria. One way of conducting this analysis is to have team members "vote" on the extent in which the vendor's pump meets RFP criteria. Cards with the numbers 1–4 can be handed out to team members. Team members who vote "1" indicate that the pump has poor performance according to criteria. Team members who vote "2" indicate that the pump has adequate, but sub-optimal, performance according to the criteria. A vote of "3" indicates that the pump meets criteria, and "4" indicates that the pump exceeds the criteria. Voting cards are held up all at once; the team members look at others' votes, and achieves consensus on the final vote. This is done over again for each of the criteria present in the RFP. Vendors who score highest by consensus are invited to the site for a demonstration visit. The RFP process will allow the team to pick a select number of vendors who meet essential criteria. This select number of vendors will then be asked to provide more detailed information and to present their product to the team. A site visit will

1. Overview

1.1. Intent

This is a Request for Proposal (RFP) by our company, is a contractual agreement to purchase pumps (large volume, PCA, syringe, and epidural) and sets for affiliated hospital sites and clinics.

1.2. Goals and Objectives

Project Goals are:
- Identify clinical needs system wide and define essential criteria.
- Explore currently available infusion pump technology and compare to criteria.
- Identify market options that maximize patient outcomes, patient safety and staff efficiency, while also minimizing variation system wide.

1.3. Our Company

Describe "our company" and the work that it does. This may include your mission, vision, values, strategic initiatives, financial, and operating performance.

1.4. Term of Agreement

List time periods that you expect to make purchases.

2. Scope of Service: Our Company Entities

2.1. The Scope of Service includes the following entities:

- Hospital #1 (350 beds)
- Hospital #2 (400 beds)
- Also include clinics and infusion centers

3. Invitation to Bid and Response Instructions

3.1. Invitation

Vendors are invited to submit proposals on equipment and supplies that are currently FDA approved and available on the marketplace. Proposed purchase shall include:
- Large volume pumps
- PCA/pain management pumps
- Syringe pumps
- Epidural pumps
- IV sets

3.2. Schedule for RFP

List deadline for submission of questions, deadline for submission of RFP, timeline for vendor presentations, and timeline for decision-making.

Proposal Response Format
- Specific detail in responses is essential for differentiation of competitive products. (Example: Criteria: Infusion rates 0.1–50.0 mL/hr. An acceptable response would be "0.1–100.0 mL/hr." An unacceptable response would be "yes.")

Continued

Figure 2-1. Sample RFP.

3.3.   Award Basis

Our company has determined that the following criteria will be used to evaluate the responses from all vendors:
*   The ability to meet goals and objectives noted
*   Ability to meet critical criteria
*   Total cost
*   Vendor organization and experience

RFP Responses: Vendor will supply the following information:

3.4.   General Information Regarding the Vendor Company

3.4.1. History

Date founded and history of company.

3.4.2. Regional Office

Identify location of health care regional office, with listing of personnel assigned to that office and company function.

3.4.3. Financial Statements

Include your most current audited financial statement for full year operation. If Company is a subsidiary of another corporation, some information must be provided for parent company.

3.5.   Experience and References of Staff Providing Services

Vendors must include an attachment that lists current accounts similarly sized to our hospitals that use the equipment offered. References should include the site location, the bed size of the site, length of time equipment has been in use and a contact person at the site who manages the area using the equipment.

3.6.   Support Training and Development Program

Vendors must include an outline of support training and development programs available to staff, including any on-going support as needed.

3.7.   Warranty (Original) and Extended

Vendors must indicate the length of time the original manufacturer's warranty will be honored. Warranty time will begin on the date of first successful patient use.

3.8.   Trade-In/Conversion Program Options

Vendors should propose all available options relating to the existing equipment. Various alternatives requested include:
*   Trade-in quotations on owned equipment
*   Updating existing equipment

3.9.   Additional Information Request

3.9.1. Delivery/Freight Charge

Vendors should consider in their proposals their terms of delivery.

Continued

Figure 2-1 (cont'd). Sample RFP.

3.9.2. Additional Information

Submit at least one example of each of the following:
- Failure mode effects analysis
- How your company incorporates human factors into the pump design process

4. Requirements of Contract

4.1. Term

Time frame during which the agreement is expected to take place.

4.2. Pricing and Alternative Pricing Proposals

Time period during which the proposed price is in effect.

4.3. Future Increase

Conditions under which the price may increase, after the initial contract period (typically based on the medical CPI for the region).

4.4. Contractual Problems/Cancellation of Contract

How will the vendor be notified of problems and a potential contract cancellation? (For example, a verbal warning, a 30-day notice, or a 60-day notice.)

Figure 2-1 (cont'd). Sample RFP.

Table 2-1. Desirable Features of Infusion Pumps

Large Volume Pumps	PCA Management Pumps	Syringe Pumps	Epidural Pumps
General Pump Requirements			
Both single and triple channel pump options available	N/A	N/A	Pump designated as epidural/intrathecal use only
2- and 4-channel pump options available	N/A	N/A	N/A
Can infuse 4 channels simultaneously	N/A	N/A	N/A
Able to infuse channels into separate or the same IV line	N/A	N/A	N/A
Modular system	Modular system	Modular system	Modular system
IV tubing/pump sets are nonproprietary and interchangeable between models	IV tubing/pump sets are nonproprietary and interchangeable between models	IV tubing/pump sets are nonproprietary and interchangeable between models	IV tubing/pump sets are interchangeable between models

Continued

Table 2-1. Desirable Features of Infusion Pumps (cont'd)

Large Volume Pumps	PCA Management Pumps	Syringe Pumps	Epidural Pumps
N/A	Specific tubing for PCA use only (visual cue/color-coded)	N/A	Dedicated tubing sets for epidural use only (visual cue/color-coded)
	PCA-designated tubing with no injection ports	N/A	Epidural-designated tubing with no injection ports
N/A	Can accommodate either bags or syringes	N/A	Can accommodate either bags or syringes
N/A	Accommodates all syringe sizes 1-60 mL	Accommodates all syringe sizes 1-60 mL	
N/A	Will accept commercially available pre-filled syringes from multiple vendors (if syringe-based)	N/A	Epidural/intrathecal tubing only compatible with epidural/IT catheters; prevents IV tubing misconnections
N/A	Correctly identifies syringe size and vendor (for syringe-based delivery)	Correctly identifies syringe size and vendor (for syringe-based delivery)	
Basic Pump Operation/Programming			
Flow rate 0.1–999 mL/hr	N/A	Infusion rates 0.01–100 mL/hr	Infusion rates 0.1–50 mL/hr
Calibrated in tenths of mL	N/A	Requires programming to four decimal places (0.0001)	
Flow rate up to 4000 mL/hr	N/A	N/A	N/A
Flow accuracy ± 5%	Flow accuracy ± 5%	Flow accuracy ± 5%	Flow accuracy ± 5%
"Keep open" rate as low as 1 mL/hr; KVO rate programmable	N/A	N/A	N/A
Continuous flow technology	Continuous flow technology	Continuous flow technology	Continuous flow technology
N/A	N/A	Ability to deliver medication "IV push"	N/A
Easy-to-read screen	Easy-to-read screen	Easy-to-read screen	Easy-to-read screen
Adjustable back light	Adjustable back light	Adjustable back light	Adjustable back light

Continued

Table 2-1. Desirable Features of Infusion Pumps [cont'd]

Large Volume Pumps	PCA Management Pumps	Syringe Pumps	Epidural Pumps
Easy to program and load tubing	Easy to program and load tubing	Easy to program and load tubing	Easy to program and load tubing
Can view entire program on one screen before activating flow	Can view entire program on one screen before activating flow	Can view entire program on one screen before activating flow	Can view entire program on one screen before activating flow
Front panel/screen lockout to preserve settings	Front panel/screen lockout to preserve settings	Front panel/screen lockout to preserve settings	Front panel/screen lockout to preserve settings
Double stroke/ double bump safety feature	Double stroke/ double bump safety feature	Double stroke/ double bump safety feature	Double stroke/ double bump safety feature
Standby mode (allows waiting period after programming, without alarming)	Standby mode (allows waiting period after programming, without alarming)	Standby mode (allows waiting period after programming, without alarming)	Standby mode (allows waiting period after programming, without alarming)
"Program retention" retains settings indefinitely but "forces choice" between current and "new" settings when turned on	"Program retention" retains settings indefinitely but "forces choice" between current and "new" settings when turned on	"Program retention" retains settings indefinitely but "forces choice" between current and "new" settings when turned on	"Program retention" retains settings indefinitely but "forces choice" between current and "new" settings when turned on
Automatic retention of programmed settings for at least 5 hours	Automatic retention of programmed settings for at least 5 hours	Automatic retention of programmed settings for at least 5 hours	Automatic retention of programmed settings for at least 5 hours
"Pause/standby" feature allows 60 second pause (for troubleshooting, blood draws) without losing programmed settings or alarming	"Pause/standby" feature allows 60 second pause (for troubleshooting, blood draws) without losing programmed settings or alarming	"Pause/standby" feature allows 60 second pause (for troubleshooting, blood draws) without losing programmed settings or alarming	"Pause/standby" feature allows 60 second pause (for troubleshooting, blood draws) without losing programmed settings or alarming
Set-based freeflow protection/anti free-flow protection if tubing removed from pump	Set-based freeflow protection if drug is bag-based	N/A	Bag-based freeflow protection
Ability to lock/secure medication bag	Ability to lock/secure medication bag	Ability to lock/secure medication bag	Ability to lock/secure medication bag
Prefer no door over tubing	Bag/label must remain visible when secured	Syringe/label must remain visible during infusion	Syringe/label must remain visible during infusion

Continued

Table 2-1. Desirable Features of Infusion Pumps (cont'd)

Large Volume Pumps	PCA Management Pumps	Syringe Pumps	Epidural Pumps
Pump attaches to IV pole	Attaches to pole; locking mechanism	Attaches to pole; locking mechanism	Attaches to pole; locking mechanism

Alarms & Indicators

Large Volume Pumps	PCA Management Pumps	Syringe Pumps	Epidural Pumps
Visual cue for infusion running	Visual cue for infusion running	Visual cue for infusion running	Visual cue for infusion running
Visual cue for infusion rate "outside range parameters" for specific drug	Visual cue for infusion rate "outside range parameters" for specific drug	Visual cue for infusion rate "outside range parameters" for specific drug	Visual cue for infusion rate "outside range parameters" for specific drug
All alarms are both audible and visible	All alarms are both audible and visible	All alarms are both audible and visible	All alarms are both audible and visible
Volume control for alarms	Volume control for alarms	Volume control for alarms	Volume control for alarms
"Silence" mode (temporarily stop alarm while troubleshooting, without losing programming)	"Silence" mode (temporarily stop alarm while troubleshooting, without losing programming)	"Silence" mode (temporarily stop alarm while troubleshooting, without losing programming)	"Silence" mode (temporarily stop alarm while troubleshooting, without losing programming)
"Abandon" alarm (if left in programming mode)	"Abandon" alarm (if left in programming mode)	"Abandon" alarm (if left in programming mode)	"Abandon" alarm (if left in programming mode)
Upstream and downstream occlusion alarms	Upstream and downstream occlusion alarms	Downstream occlusion alarm	Upstream and downstream occlusion alarms (M)
Adjustable occlusion pressures (programmable to match library)	Adjustable occlusion pressures (programmable to match library)	Adjustable occlusion pressures (programmable to match library)	Adjustable occlusion pressures (programmable to match library)
"30 second occlusion re-set" (does not alarm if problem self-resolves in 30 seconds)	"30 second occlusion re-set" (does not alarm if problem self-resolves in 30 seconds)	"30 second occlusion re-set" (does not alarm if problem self-resolves in 30 seconds)	"30 second occlusion re-set" (does not alarm if problem self-resolves in 30 seconds)
"Air in line" alarm	"Air in line" alarm	N/A	"Air in line" alarm
"Empty line" alarm	"Empty line" alarm	N/A	"Empty line" alarm
"Infusion complete" alarm for empty IV or programmed amount complete	"Infusion complete" alarm for empty IV or programmed amount complete	"Infusion complete" alarm for empty IV or programmed amount complete	"Infusion complete" alarm for empty IV or programmed amount complete
"Dry drip chamber" alarm (alarms prior to being empty; not reported as "upstream occlusion")	N/A	"Smart" alarm for "near empty" (calculates 5–30 minutes remaining)	"Smart" alarm for "near empty" (calculates 5–30 minutes remaining)

Continued

Table 2-1. Desirable Features of Infusion Pumps (cont'd)

Large Volume Pumps	PCA Management Pumps	Syringe Pumps	Epidural Pumps
Alarm for "secondary infusion" not infusing	N/A	N/A	N/A
"Secondary infusion complete" alarm	N/A	N/A	N/A
"Secondary infusion occlusion" alarm	N/A	N/A	N/A
"Smart Pump" Requirements			
Drug/Dose standards with hard and soft dosing limits	Drug/Dose standards with hard and soft dosing limits	Drug/Dose standards with hard and soft dosing limits	Drug/Dose standards with hard and soft dosing limits
Dose delivery available in several modes (i.e. mL/hr, mg/min, mcg/min, mcg/kg/min, units/hr)	Dosing in mg or mcg	Dose delivery in several modes, including weight-based calculations (e.g., "units/kg/hr") and "bolus" dose option with specific limits	Dose delivery only in mL
N/A	Able to program individual doses and continuous/basal infusion rate	Infusion rate based on drug calculation and syringe size	N/A
N/A	Able to program higher doses for basal infusion rates (>100 mcg/hr)	N/A	N/A
N/A	PCA doses supported by pump	N/A	N/A
"Keep open" rate programmable with library	N/A	N/A	N/A
Minimum of 10 drug libraries with weight range (in kg) for each	Minimum of 6 drug libraries with weight range (in kg) for each	Minimum of 6 drug libraries with weight range (in kg) for each	Minimum of 2 drug libraries with weight range (in kg) for each
100 drug capacity for each library	10 drug capacity for each library	32–64 drug capacity for each library	20 drug capacity for each library
Options for accessing multiple libraries with each pump	Options for accessing multiple libraries with each pump	Options for accessing multiple libraries with each pump	Options for accessing multiple libraries with each pump
When using multiple channels, drug program prevents infusing same drug in more than one line	N/A	N/A	N/A

Continued

Table 2-1. Desirable Features of Infusion Pumps (cont'd)

Large Volume Pumps	PCA Management Pumps	Syringe Pumps	Epidural Pumps
No "Do Not Use" abbreviations used in library	No "Do Not Use" abbreviations used in library	No "Do Not Use" abbreviations used in library	No "Do Not Use" abbreviations used in library
Allows use of "TALL man" lettering for medications	Allows use of "TALL man" lettering for medications	Allows use of "TALL man" lettering for medications	Allows use of "TALL man" lettering for medications
System defaults to dose error reduction system upon start-up	System defaults to dose error reduction system upon start-up	System defaults to dose error reduction system upon start-up	System defaults to dose error reduction system upon start-up
Weights must have ranges appropriate to patient population	Weights must have ranges appropriate to patient population	Weights must have ranges appropriate to patient population	Weights must have ranges appropriate to patient population
Allows soft and hard weight limits to be set within each library	Allows soft and hard weight limits to be set within each library	Allows soft and hard weight limits to be set within each library	Allows soft and hard weight limits to be set within each library
Allows facility to require confirmation of weight entry	Allows facility to require confirmation of weight entry	Allows facility to require confirmation of weight entry	Allows facility to require confirmation of weight entry
Programs for calculations in Kg	Programs for calculations must be in Kg	Programs for calculations must be in Kg	Programs for calculations must be in Kg

Dose Error Reduction System/Electronic Interface

Maintains "event history" > 500 events (key presses, error codes, alarms, amount infused)	Maintains "event history" > 500 events (key presses, error codes, alarms, amount infused)	Maintains "event history" > 500 events (key presses, error codes, alarms, amount infused)	Maintains "event history" > 500 events (key presses, error codes, alarms, amount infused)
Maintains "event history" for 5+ hours	Maintains "event history" for 5+ hours	Maintains "event history" for 5+ hours	Maintains "event history" for 5+ hours
Able to download event history electronically	Able to download event history electronically	Able to download event history electronically	Able to download event history electronically
Wireless upload/ download of information	Wireless upload/ download of information	Wireless upload/ download of information	Wireless upload/ download of information
Two-way wireless interface with electronic medical record	Two-way wireless interface with electronic medical record	Two-way wireless interface with electronic medical record	Two-way wireless interface with electronic medical record

Continued

Table 2-1. Desirable Features of Infusion Pumps (cont'd)

Large Volume Pumps	PCA Management Pumps	Syringe Pumps	Epidural Pumps
Barcode reading capability for medication	Barcode reading capability for medication	Barcode reading capability for medication	Barcode reading capability for medication
Has capability to revise/upgrade software (prefer wireless uploading capability)	Has capability to revise/upgrade software (prefer wireless uploading capability)	Has capability to revise/upgrade software (prefer wireless uploading capability)	Has capability to revise/upgrade software (prefer wireless uploading capability)
Power Source/Battery			
Operates long-term on AC	Operates long-term on AC or battery	Operates long-term on AC	Operates long-term on AC or battery
Full operation 4+ hours on single battery charge	Full operation 4+ hours on single battery charge	Full operation 4+ hours on single battery charge	Full operation 4+ hours on single battery charge
Provides "low battery" warning with 30 minutes remaining and retains programming	Provides "low battery" warning with 30 minutes remaining and retains programming	Provides "low battery" warning with 30 minutes remaining and retains programming	Provides "low battery" warning with 30 minutes remaining and retains programming
Residual memory (maintains drug library if battery totally depleted)	Residual memory (maintains drug library if battery totally depleted)	Residual memory (maintains drug library if battery totally depleted)	Residual memory (maintains drug library if battery totally depleted)
Visual indicator for level of battery charge remaining	Visual indicator for level of battery charge remaining	Visual indicator for level of battery charge remaining	Visual indicator for level of battery charge remaining
Recovery time to full battery charge < 4 hours	Recovery time to full battery charge < 4 hours	Recovery time to full battery charge < 4 hours	Recovery time to full battery charge < 4 hours
Battery life 12 months minimum; not shortened by battery completely discharging	Battery life 12 months minimum; not shortened by battery completely discharging	Battery life 12 months minimum; not shortened by battery completely discharging	Battery life 12 months minimum; not shortened by battery completely discharging
No transformer in power cord	No transformer in power cord	No transformer in power cord	No transformer in power cord
Cord permanently attached to back of pump	Cord detaches from pump	Cord detaches from pump	Cord detaches from pump
Cord length 10 ft	Cord length 10 ft	Cord length 10 ft	Cord length 10 ft
Securing mechanism for cord (quick, easy, secure) during patient transport	Securing mechanism for cord (quick, easy, secure) during patient transport	Securing mechanism for cord (quick, easy, secure) during patient transport	Securing mechanism for cord (quick, easy, secure) during patient transport

Continued

Table 2-1. Desirable Features of Infusion Pumps (cont'd)

Large Volume Pumps	PCA Management Pumps	Syringe Pumps	Epidural Pumps
Miscellaneous			
N/A	ET CO2 monitoring feedback	N/A	Same as PCA pump
N/A	Oximetry monitoring feedback	N/A	Same as PCA pump
N/A	PCA button secures to pump	N/A	N/A
N/A	PCA button is restricted to use by the patient or nurse via bio-ID or other method	N/A	Option for PCEA (patient-controlled epidural anesthesia therapy)
ECRI rating is "recommended" in an assessment performed within the past 36 months	ECRI rating is "recommended" in an assessment performed within the past 36 months	ECRI rating is "recommended" in an assessment performed within the past 36 months	ECRI rating is "recommended" in an assessment performed within the past 36 months
Education/Service/Vendor Support			
Vendor education support during conversion and ongoing			
DVD or online resources to assist in clinical competency development			
Local field service support			
Provide the Following Information for Each Pump and Model			
Tubing/sets: What brands of tubing are compatible with your pump?	Tubing/sets: What brands of tubing are compatible with your pump?	Tubing/sets: What brands of tubing are compatible with your pump?	Tubing/sets: What brands of tubing are compatible with your pump?
Specify dimensions and weight of each pump model	Specify dimensions and weight of each pump model	Specify dimensions and weight of each pump model	Specify dimensions and weight of each pump model
Describe process for initial drug library programming and subsequent updating	Describe process for initial drug library programming and subsequent updating	Describe process for initial drug library programming and subsequent updating	Describe process for initial drug library programming and subsequent updating
Specify how pumps are cleaned (spray on disinfectant, wipe off or other)	Specify how pumps are cleaned (spray on disinfectant, wipe off or other)	Specify how pumps are cleaned (spray on disinfectant, wipe off or other)	Specify how pumps are cleaned (spray on disinfectant, wipe off or other)

Continued

Large Volume Pumps	PCA Management Pumps	Syringe Pumps	Epidural Pumps
Table 2-1. Desirable Features of Infusion Pumps (cont'd)			
Specify routine maintenance requirements	Specify routine maintenance requirements	Specify routine maintenance requirements	Specify routine maintenance requirements

include the vendor's presentation of the pump itself, along with a presentation of the future vision of the company. After the vendor presentation, team members are allowed to "play" with the pump to gauge whether responses to criteria in the RFP are accurate. Final scoring of the vendors for meeting criteria is again done. The RFP process, while time-consuming, can help the team clarify which vendors will most likely meet the needs of the health system, thereby saving time in the long run.

The evaluation of the supplier's goods and services may also be evaluated with a tool called the value analysis process. The value of an item is determined by estimating how well it performs, divided by the cost of the item. Value analysis[1] is a systematic, objective process for evaluating and reducing supply expenses by considering alternate products and practices. Product selected must meet the needs of the institution while maintaining or improving quality of care. Value analysis is a customer focused, process oriented, and data-driven. The thing that differentiates value analysis from an ordinary RFP is the fact that cost of the product is included in the analysis. Cost is taken into consideration, along with product performance. Costs may be given equal weight to product performance.

In order to conduct the value analysis, the team "weighted" the pump criteria, according to the importance of each feature. A weighted decision making matrix was developed by group consensus. This weighted matrix recognizes that certain attributes absolutely must be present, while other attributes are only listed as desirable. A larger numerical weighting means that the attribute is highly desired or critical to the pump. If an object performs exceptionally well in an attribute with a high matrix value, it is thought to provide more value overall.

Each attribute category was weighted on a score of one to ten. Sub-category criteria were also weighted. For example, one category was entitled "the quality of clinical/technical education, training, and consultation." Total category weight was 10 (highest possible value). Subcategories of this category and their weighting included "vendor is able to provide education and support during conversion and ongoing as requested" (weight = 6), "vendor offers regularly scheduled continuing education as requested" (weight = 1), and "vendor provides multimedia educational tools to assist in clinical staff competency development" (weight = 3). Notice that the subcategory weightings add up to the total weighting for this category (6 + 1+ 3 = 10). An example of a weighted decision matrix is in Table 2-2.

Suppliers responded through the RFP process and presented information to the selection team. Suppliers were given one hour to conduct a formal presentation to the selection team using media presentations and pump demonstrations. Suppliers were then asked to set up booths at which team members could get hands-on experience with the pumps and ask questions. Team members used a weighted decision making matrix, hands-on clinical simulations, and human factors usability evaluations. In the weighted decision matrix, each category and sub-category was given a score between one and four. The score was multiplied by the weighting to obtain an overall total score, allowing for comparisons between the pumps. General points of selection considerations are represented in Table 2-3.

The end result of this process is to identify any pumps that did not meet critical criteria for our health system. The pumps that were successful in meeting critical criteria would go on to the next step in the process, which was failure modes and effects analysis and usability testing, described in Chapter 3.

Table 2-2. Sample Weighted Decision Matrix

Attribute	Weight of Attribute (Range 1–10)	Attribute Score for Pump #1 (Range 1–4)	Total Weighted Score for Pump #1 (Weight × Score)	Attribute Score for Pump #2 (Range 1–4)	Total Weighted Score for Pump #2 (Weight × Score)
Vendor is able to provide ongoing education after implementation	6	4	24	2	12
Vendor offers continuing education	1	2	2	4	4
Vendor provides multimedia education tools	3	1	3	3	9
			Total score for pump #1 = 29		Total score for pump #2 = 25

In this example above, pump #1 is rated higher than pump #2, even though pump #2 scored higher in two of the attributes. The team gave the education after implementation attribute a higher value; pump #1 scored higher in that attribute and therefore is more highly rated.

Conclusion

A well-planned and well-executed pump selection process is critical to the success of the vendor selection process. The most important members of the team are the bedside caregivers, who can give valuable feedback on the utility of the pump in "real life" situations. Communication of the vendor selection process is also critical to a successful implementation.

Table 2-3. Smart Pump Selection Assessment Points

General

- Estimated number of smart pumps to be purchased or leased
- Type of smart pumps (IV, PCA, syringe) needed
- Patient population (adult/peds)
- Estimated number of drug labels needed in library
- Estimated number of clinical areas for use
- Line utilization (single-channel, double-channel, etc.)

Technology

- Bar-coding point of care capable
- CPOE capable
- Electronic medication administration record capabilities
- Pharmacy information system
- Medication dispensing cabinets
- The organization's future technology implementation projects

Outcomes/Data Collection

- Wireless or manual download capabilities
- Outcome measures

Implementation

- Infrastructure upgrades
- Technological upgrades/purchases (software/networks required)
- Staff training/education

Financial

- Estimated smart pump budget
  - Cost of smart pumps
  - Cost of administration sets
  - Cost of service contract

Vendor Relations

- Interview/clinical simulation
- Service/maintenance (onsite/emergency support) performance
- Initial/ongoing staff training
- Future system upgrades planned
- References from organizations using vendor's pumps

PRACTICE TIPS

- Make sure that other components of pump utilization are included in your analysis. Examples of these include the cost of pump rental, costs of cleaning fluids, IV tubing, IV solutions contracts, and ready-to-use products such as Vial Mate® and Mini Bag Plus®.
- A change in pumps may also mean a change in IV solutions and nutritionals. This is a major change process in itself. A crosswalk should be developed to map old solutions to comparable new solutions. The solution content may not be exactly the same. The crosswalk should include purchase item numbers and be distributed to both pharmacy buyers and materials management staff. Decisions should be made regarding the department purchasing and stocking the solutions, whether it will be the pharmacy department or materials management. Since the appearance and content of the solutions may change, a nursing communication plan should be developed.
- A change in pumps may also mean a change in tubing. Nurses will need education regarding the use and appearance of the new tubing. If there is different tubing for gravity flow versus pump flow? Be sure that the gravity flow tubing will allow high flow rates that may be required in areas such as surgery, Emergency Department, and oncology infusion areas. If high flow rates cannot be used with the gravity tubing, pump tubing will be used instead, incurring higher costs.
- The pump rental process is a very important aspect of any pump implementation. Ask your vendor for a specific process on renting additional pumps. If the chosen pump has a relatively short battery life, and patients unplug the pump for extended periods of time, this will mean the pump will need to be re-charged. Re-charging the battery can be a time consuming process, resulting in pumps out of service and rentals more frequently than expected. Your biomedical services will need to take line utilization into consideration. For example, how many double-channel pumps are currently in utilization with only one line used? Data may need to be collected to discover your true line utilization.
- Simple ergonomics are important. What does the pump weigh? Can the nurse easily attach and detach the pump from the pole with their dominant hand? Does the pump slide when attached to chrome IV poles? To answer these questions, nurses really need an opportunity to "play" with the pump *prior* to pump selection.
- Ask about the cleaning solutions needed for the pump.

- Team members should be able to articulate the process of pump selection. Since you can't please everyone, there will likely be numerous questions regarding how the pump selection took place.

- Information services are key to a successful implementation. Each new wireless application launched by the organization will increase the complexity of the wireless environment. Simple configuration changes in your mobile wireless communication devices, for example, can impact on the wireless capability of the pumps.

Managing Your Vendor Relationship

- Establish expectations for communication early in the process. Weekly meetings or conference calls with the multi-disciplinary team should be an expectation.

- Ask your vendor for names of references from sites that have implemented the pump. Call the references and ask questions regarding ease of pump implementation, wireless updates, and vendor support.

- Ask how many pumps can be updated at one time, using the wireless technology. You will need to understand precisely how long it will take for the pump library update to take, since this will impact on your staffing requirements.

- Search the MAUDE database for any recalls that have occurred with the pump. Ask what actions are being taken to address the technology issues.

- Ask your vendor to share experiences from other pump implementations they have done.

- Try to stick to your commitments and timelines as closely as possible. Having timelines and deliverables laid out ahead of time will better define expectations.

Suggested Reading

Healthcare product comparison system, large volume infusion pumps, ambulatory infusion pumps, patient-controlled analgesia infusion pumps, and syringe infusion pumps. ECRI Institute. Available at: www.ecri.org/documents/HPCS_Infusion_Pumps.pdf

Smart Pumps 2008. KLAS Enterprises, LLC. Subscription required.

References

1. Bennatan EM. *Software Project Management.* 2nd ed. New York: McGraw-Hill International; 1992.

2. Miles LD. Techniques of value analysis and engineering. Madison, WI: Wendt Library. Available at: http://wendt.library.wisc.edu/miles/milesbook.html. Accessed February 25, 2009.

Human Factors Testing to Aid in the Selection of Intravenous Infusion Pumps:

Usability Testing and Failure Modes and Effects Analysis

Kathleen A. Harder and John R. Bloomfield

Key Terms

Failure modes and effects analysis (FMEA)—a process by which potential failures of a device or system are uncovered.

Human factors techniques—the study of human interaction with devices, processes, and systems.

Usability testing—a test to determine how well a device functions in a real-life scenario.

Introduction

There are two human factors techniques that should play an important part in the selection of medical devices, such as intravenous infusion pumps. The techniques are—(1) usability testing, and (2) failure modes and effects analysis (FMEA).

Usability testing is conducted to evaluate a system or device. In a usability test, the system or device is tested in a controlled situation by potential users, in order to obtain information on how well the device or system is likely to perform in the environment for which it is intended.

An FMEA is a procedure that is used to discover potential failure modes in a system or device. Potential failures may occur because of deficiencies or flaws in the system or device, and/or because of the way in which it is used. In addition to uncovering potential failures, an FMEA will also indicate the effects that the potential failures might have.

The way in which usability testing and the FMEA should be used to test infusion pumps is discussed in the following sections of this chapter.

Usability Testing

Pre-Test Selection of Pumps

Before conducting a usability test of infusion pumps, the manufacturer's information on the candidate pumps should be examined and evaluated critically by a group representing the purchasing organization. It is important that this group includes nurses who will use infusion pumps to treat patients; the nurses should be drawn from a range of nursing practice areas—e.g., emergency department, obstetrics, pediatrics, medsurg, the PACU, NICU, PICU, Adult ICU, Oncology, Peds BMT, and Adult BMT. They should be drawn from a wide range of practice areas because the needs of the nursing staff may vary considerably from one practice area to another. The initial critical examination and evaluation should be conducted in order to identify those pumps that have the features that are required by the purchasing organization.

After the pumps with the required features have been identified, a usability test can be conducted to determine how well each of the identified pumps performs in practice. For a usability test, it is advisable to limit the number of pumps that are to be tested to three or four—otherwise the test may become unwieldy.

Method

Participants
If possible, there should be 20 or more participants in the usability study. These participants should:

- Have varying amounts of experience—e.g., perhaps half of them should have provided acute care/inpatient nursing care for from one to 10 years, while the remaining half should have provided acute care/inpatient nursing care for more than 10 years.
- Be drawn from a wide range of facilities operated by the purchasing organization, so that the potentially diverse range of user needs will be represented during the usability test.
- Represent a range of nursing practice areas. In addition to sampling nursing staff from the areas represented in the initial selection phase (e.g., the emergency department, obstetrics, pediatrics, medsurg, the PACU, NICU, PICU, adult ICU, oncology, peds BMT, and adult BMT) there should participants from the float pool.

Test Set-up
To illustrate how the usability test should be conducted, we will assume that four large volume IV pumps will be evaluated—e.g., Pump A, Pump B, Pump C, and Pump D. At least two of each of the pumps should be present at the usability test site. One of each of the four pumps should be located in a separate test room. Thus there will be four test rooms, each containing one of the pumps

that will be evaluated in the usability test. The second pump of each type (A, B, C, and D) should be located in an area in which participants can briefly (e.g., 15 minutes) familiarize themselves with the pumps before testing them in the dedicated test rooms.

In the familiarization area, the participants will be able to briefly work with each pump and use the educational materials provided by the manufacturer of each pump.

Instructions to Participants

During the usability test, the participants should be instructed not to discuss the pumps with each other. They should be told that observers are noting how the pumps function while the participants use them—that they are not observing the participants themselves. After each step, the participants should tell the observer that they have finished the step. They should also be told that if they cannot complete one of the steps, they should tell the observer and then move on to the next step. They should then complete an evaluation for the pump.

Controlling for Effects of Order

Again, assuming that four pumps are to be evaluated, each participant should be assigned to one of four groups. When the participants from each group evaluate the pumps, they should visit the test rooms in a prescribed order. There should be a different order for each group—and the four orders should be counterbalanced. Counterbalancing minimizes potential effects of order. If potential effects of order are not controlled for with counterbalancing (i.e., if all participants evaluate the pumps in the same order), it is possible that the participant's experience with the first pump could affect the participant's evaluation of the second pump, which in turn could affect his/her evaluation of the third pump, and so on; the effect of one pump's evaluation on the next would make data interpretation problematic. The order in which the participants evaluate the pumps can be counterbalanced by using a Latin square. Table 3-1 presents an example of a counterbalanced order.

Table 3-1. Typical Counterbalanced Order for Testing Four Pumps

Group 1	Pump A	Pump C	Pump B	Pump D
Group 2	Pump C	Pump D	Pump A	Pump B
Group 3	Pump B	Pump A	Pump D	Pump C
Group 4	Pump D	Pump B	Pump C	Pump A

A Latin square, like the one shown in Table 3-1, is an *n* x *n* table in which *n* different symbols are arranged in such a way that each symbol occurs just once in each row and once in each column. In addition, the Latin square used in Table 3-1 has an added property—i.e., each symbol (which, in this case represents one of the four infusion pumps) is preceded and followed by each other symbol only once. Twenty-four unique Latin squares can be obtained with four symbols; however, only 6 of these 24 Latin squares have the property of having each symbol preceded and followed by each other symbol only once. See Figure 3-1.

A Latin square is an *n* x *n* table in which *n* different symbols are arranged in such a way that each symbol occurs just once in each row and in each column. When *n = 4*, there are 24 possible unique Latin squares when four symbols are arranged so that each symbol occurs just once in each row and once in each column. However, only 6 of these 24 Latin squares have the additional property whereby each symbol is preceded and followed by each other symbol only once. These six Latin squares are presented below. The example given in the main text is Latin square #3.

Latin Square #1

A	B	C	D
B	D	A	C
C	A	D	B
D	C	B	A

Latin Square #4

A	C	D	B
C	B	A	D
B	D	C	A
D	A	B	C

Latin Square #2

A	B	D	C
B	C	A	D
C	D	B	A
D	A	C	B

Latin Square #5

A	D	B	C
D	C	A	B
B	A	C	D
C	B	D	A

Latin Square #3

A	C	B	D
C	D	A	B
B	A	D	C
D	B	C	A

Latin Square #6

A	D	C	B
D	B	A	C
B	C	D	A
C	A	B	D

Figure 3-1. Latin squares (with four symbols).

Process

Each participant should begin by briefly familiarizing him- or herself with each of the pumps to be tested—working with the pump and any available educational materials. Then, each participant should visit the test rooms and test the different pumps in the order prescribed for their group. While working in the room assigned for each pump, the participants should use the pump to carry out a scripted scenario derived from normal clinical practice. The same scenario should be used for all four different pumps. An example of such a scripted scenario derived from normal clinical practice is presented in Figure 3-2.

Immediately after finishing his or her session with each pump, the participant should complete a survey pertaining to his or her perceptions of that pump. This survey should ask each participant: (1) to rate how easy was it for him or her to program the pump overall; (2) whether or not he or she thought that the pump's programming sequence was logical; (3) to rate how easy it was for him or her to

An example of two scripted scenarios derived from normal clinical practice is presented below:

Patient A:

- Order reads: 1000 D5 ½ NS with 20 KCl @ 100 mL/hr.
- Increase rate to 125 mL/hr.
- Place pump on hold.
- Add Ceftaz 1 gram in 50 mL to infuse over 10 minutes.
- Using a second channel/pump: Lipids 20% @ 5 mL/hr x 20 hours (100 mL total)
- Program maintenance fluid to run 500 mL (D5 ½ NS) over 30 minutes.
- Stop infusion and reduce rate to 10 mL/hr.
- Turn pump off. Turn pump back on and resume same settings for Patient A.
- Begin Levophed 4 mg/250 cc @ 2 mcg/min.
- Activate "Lock Out" feature.
- Turn pump off.

Patient B: (weight 14 kg)

Using the smart pump feature:
- Run dopamine @ 5 mcg/kg/min for a 14 kg patient using standard concentration dopamine 400 mg in 250 ml.
- Titrate up to 6 mcg/kg/min for a brief time.
- Titrate down to 3 mcg/kg/min for a brief time.
- Titrate up to 36 mcg/kg/min.
- Change concentration to—320 mg in 50 mL.
- Program a secondary infusion of Rocephin 1 gram in 50 mL on this line.

Figure 3-2. Scripted scenarios for a usability test of infusion pumps.

follow the pump cues; (4) if he or she noticed a programming mistake, to rate how easy was it for him or her to identify that mistake; (5) if he or she made a programming mistake, to rate how easy was it for him or her to correct that mistake; (6) considering font size, legibility, and glare (if any), to rate how easy was it for him or her to read the information on the pump display; (7) to rate how confident he or she is that the pump will do what it was programmed to do; and (8) to rate the extent to which he or she liked or disliked the pump. Participants will be asked to use a 7-point category scale to rate their response to questions about each pump. An example of a survey is presented in Appendix 3-1.

After completing his or her evaluation of a pump, the participant should move on to the next room and pump in the prescribed order.

Observers

During the usability testing there should be four objective observers, with one observer assigned to each pump test room. The role of each observer is to watch how the participants work with the pump in the test room. The observers should be instructed not to provide any help or information to any participant; the observers are *not* in the pump test room to coach the participants. After watching each participant testing the pump, the observer should rate the pump on the following dimensions: (1) how easy was it for the participant to program the pump overall; (2) how easy was it for the participant to identify a programming mistake; (3) how easy was it for the participant to correct a programming mistake. The observers should also use a seven-point rating scale to indicate their ratings. Each observer should provide ratings after each participant has worked with the particular pump to which the observer is assigned. An example of the observer's scoring sheet is presented in Appendix 3-2.

Results

Typically, it will be possible to use an analysis of variance (ANOVA) to compare the ratings obtained from participants who are exposed to all of the pumps tested in a usability test. The ANOVA will indicate whether or not there are statistically significant differences in the responses obtained for the different pumps. If there are significant differences, an appropriate *post hoc* test, like the Fisher's PLSD test or the Tukey-Kramer test, can be used to make pairwise comparisons and determine which specific pumps are producing the significant differences and, also, which pump receives the statistically significant highest ratings.

It should be noted that there may be mismatches between the ratings of the participants and the ratings of the observers. These mismatches are particularly informative, and are most likely to occur with a pump that is in current use at the facilities of the purchasing organization—with the participants giving higher ratings to that pump than the observers.

The results of the usability test will provide information as to which pump is easiest to use, will be least likely to lead to medication administration errors, will enhance patient care, and will yield higher levels of patient safety.

Failure Modes and Effects Analysis

The next step in the selection process should be to conduct an FMEA on the pump(s) that emerged from the usability test as the top candidate(s). If two of the four pumps received similar usability ratings, then both should be subjected to an FMEA. The FMEA is expected to further distinguish one pump from the other. The analysis is intended to drill further down into the functionality and usability of a particular pump. Those conducting the FMEA should attempt to "break the pump" (i.e., they should determine how the pump responds to mistakes they intentionally make).

Participants

The FMEA should be conducted by a human factors expert and two or three very experienced nurses and at least one pharmacist—the nurses should come from different nursing practice areas—although in this case it is advisable to have the nurses come from areas in which IV infusion pumps are extensively used—e.g.,

ICU or BMT areas. Those who use IV infusion pumps extensively will have the expertise (skill set) needed to most effectively assess whether the pump is designed to meet their needs as they care for patients with complex problems.

Several complex scripted scenarios derived from normal clinical practice, should be used in the FMEA. Unlike the generic scenarios developed for the usability testing, the scenarios used for the FMEA should be tailored to specifically address the features and functionality of the particular pumps included in the analysis—one set of scenarios should be developed for each pump. Each scenario should be explored in detail with the testers examining the following: (1) the presentation of information (information design); (2) the way in which the pump is programmed, (3) the drug library; and (4) dosing limit functionality. As part of this testing the testers should be encouraged to make deliberate mistakes in order to determine whether or not the pump provides information to the user indicating that an error has been made, and whether or not it provides guidance on how to correct those mistakes.

Information Design

With regard to the way in which the pump presents information, the pump analyzers will explore how easy it is to understand the information presented on the screen, whether aspects of the information are difficult to understand, confusing, contradictory, or potentially misleading. Alarms and alerts should be critically examined to ensure that the desired action/message they convey will be easily comprehended by the users. If they find any problems in these areas, they will assess how the information design could be improved and how likely it would be for the current design to cause user error.

Pump Programming

With regard to programming the pump, the analyzers will determine whether or not any aspects of programming are confusing or difficult to carry out. In particular, they will explore whether or not there are any contradictions or confusions in the way that the pump has to be used in the different complex scenarios tested in the FMEA. They will determine whether there are any programming areas that are difficult to navigate, and whether there are any difficulties in shifting from one dosing regime to another. Then, they will give recommendations on potential changes in the programming functions that can be passed on to the pump manufacturers, and/or how the instructions for the users might be modified so that the problems can be anticipated and understood by the users and can be dealt with the least difficulty.

Drug Library

Organizations differ in their medication needs, so it is recommended that the drug library should have the capacity to be configured by the purchasing organization. A thorough assessment should be made to determine whether the drug library can be configured to meet both simple and complex requirements. The detailed analysis should include determining whether the user will be able to access the drug library effectively, including whether some medications will be pass code protected. The analysis should determine whether any frequently administered medications have been omitted from the drug library, and whether or not the appropriate concentrations for these medications are listed.

Limits

With regard to the limits, the testers will determine whether or not the presentation of the information regarding medication limits is easy to understand, whether or not limits are configurable by the purchasing organization, whether the limit options correspond to the limits required for the range of patients that are cared for in the facilities of the purchasing organization, and whether or not the hard and soft limits can be set appropriately for those patients. Those conducting the FMEA are expected to document recommended changes they would like to see pertaining to the way in which information regarding medication limits is presented and ask questions about whether or not the pump allows different medication limits to be configured for different patient populations (e.g., adult versus pediatric patients).

PRACTICE TIPS

- Sometimes one of the pumps, with the required features that is to be included in the usability test, may already be in current use in everyday clinical practice in the facilities of the purchasing organization. If this is the case, then the participants in the usability test will have had considerable experience with this pump—and, because of this familiarity, that particular pump is likely to have an advantage over the competing new pumps in the usability test. One way to control for this kind of familiarity effect is to have objective observers monitor the users as they test the pumps. It is advisable to have a human factors expert supervise the usability test.

- If any pump manufacturer's representatives are present at the time that the usability test is conducted, it is important that those representatives should not be allowed to interact with the participants: The point of a usability test is to determine how well a nurse can use a pump when only that pump and the instructions for it are available—not to see how well they can use a pump when a company representative is there coaching him or her.

Conclusion

This chapter describes how to utilize two human factors techniques that can play an important role in the selection of medical devices (like intravenous infusion pumps). The first of these, usability testing, provides a way to compare candidate devices under controlled conditions and employs potential users, with varying experience, as testers. The second, failure modes and effects analysis (FMEA), drills down further into the functionality of a particular device, in order to discover potential failure modes that might occur when the device is used in practice and the possible effects those failure might produce. Together, these techniques provide a systematic and rigorous analysis that will aid in the process of choosing between candidate devices, and of anticipating any problems that might be associated with them, when they are selected.

Appendix 3-1

Survey Questions for Participants in a Usability Test of Infusion Pumps

An example of a survey that could be used by the participants in a usability test for IV pumps is presented below:

<u>User Evaluation Form</u>

Note to user: Do not consult the observer, but you may use vendor resources. Please complete this feedback form after you have completed all the scenarios for this pump.

(a)   User number (assigned at sign-in) _____

(b)   State your current area of practice on the line below (e.g., ED, OB, adult medsurg, adult ICU, peds medsurg, peds ICU, OR/periop)

(c)   How long have you provided acute care/inpatient nursing care? (Please check one below.)

      < 1 year   _____
      1–10 years _____
      > 10 years _____

(d)   Pump name _____

For questions below involving a scale from 1–7, please circle a number from that best reflects your answer to the question. For example, an answer of 1 for the first question means that you think the pump was very difficult to prime and an answer of 7 means that you think the pump was very easy to prime.

A. Ease of pump set up

(1)   How easy was it for you to prime the pump?

Very difficult 1   2   3   4   5   6   7 Very easy

(2)   How easy was it for you to load the pump tubing?

Very difficult 1   2   3   4   5   6   7 Very easy

(3)   How easy was it for you to turn the pump on?

Very difficult 1   2   3   4   5   6   7 Very easy

B. Ease of programming

(4)   How easy was it for you to program the pump overall?

Very difficult 1   2   3   4   5   6   7 Very easy

(5)   Was the programming sequence logical? Yes _____ No _____

(6)   How easy was it for you to follow the pump cues?

Very difficult 1   2   3   4   5   6   7 Very easy

(7)   If you noticed that you made a programming mistake, how easy was it for you to identify it? (Do not respond to the question if it is not applicable.)

Very difficult 1   2   3   4   5   6   7 Very easy

(8)   If you made a programming mistake how easy was it for you to correct? (Do not respond to the question if it is not applicable.)

Very difficult 1   2   3   4   5   6   7 Very easy

C. Pump display

(9)   Considering font size, legibility, glare, if any, how easy was it for you to read the information on the pump display?

Very difficult 1   2   3   4   5   6   7 Very easy

(10) If you tested the pump in a dark room how easy was it for you to read the information on the pump display? (Do not respond to the question if you did not test it in a dark room.)

Very difficult 1   2   3   4   5   6   7 Very easy

D. Use of instructional aids

(11) Did you need to refer to instructional aids? Yes _____ No _____

(12) Were you able to resolve your issue(s) quickly? Yes _____ No _____

E. Additional comments, if any

_____

_____

_____

Appendix 3-2

Questions for Observers in a Usability Test of Infusion Pumps

Example of questions that should be answered by observers in a usability test for IV pumps are presented below:

<u>Observer Form—Large Volume Pump</u>

Note to observers: Please complete one feedback form for each user for each pump. It is very important that you do not offer assistance to the user. Your task is to observe, not to assist.

(a) User number: _____

(b) Pump test start time: _____

(c) Pump test stop time: _____

(d) Time to complete test: _____

(e) Type of pump: _____

(f) Pump name: _____

For questions below involving a scale from 1–7, please circle a number from that best reflects your answer to the question. For example, an answer of 1 for the first question means that you think the pump was very difficult for the user to prime and an answer of 7 means that you think it was very easy for the participant to prime the pump.

I. Ease of pump set up

(1) How easy is it for the participant to turn the pump on?

Very difficult 1   2   3   4   5   6   7 Very easy

(2) How easy is it for the user to prime the tubing?

Very difficult 1   2   3   4   5   6   7 Very easy

(3) How easy is it for the user to load the pump tubing?

Very difficult 1   2   3   4   5   6   7 Very easy

Comments _____
_____
_____
_____

II. PATIENT A

A. Ease of programming

(1) Was the pump programmed correctly? Yes _____ No _____

(2) If the pump was not programmed correctly, did the participant correct the mistake? Yes _____ No _____

(3) How easy is it for the participant to identify a programming mistake? (Do not respond to the question if it is not applicable.)

Very difficult 1   2   3   4   5   6   7 Very easy

(4) How easy is it for the participant to correct a programming mistake? (Do not respond to the question if it is not applicable.)

Very difficult 1   2   3   4   5   6   7 Very easy

(5) How easy is it for the user to program the pump overall?

Very difficult 1   2   3   4   5   6   7 Very easy

Comments _____
_____
_____
_____

B. Use of instructional aids

(6) How often did the user refer to instructional aids? (Please circle one.)

Not at all   Occasionally   Often   Very often   Constantly

(7) Was the user able to resolve his/her issue(s) quickly? Yes _____ No _____

Comments _____
_____
_____
_____

III. PATIENT B

A. Ease of programming

(1) Was the pump programmed correctly? Yes _____ No _____

(2) If the pump was not programmed correctly, did the participant correct the mistake? Yes _____ No _____

(3) How easy is it for the participant to identify a programming mistake? (Do not respond to the question if it is not applicable.)

Very difficult 1   2   3   4   5   6   7 Very easy

(4) How easy is it for the participant to correct a programming mistake? (Do not respond to the question if it is not applicable.)

Very difficult 1   2   3   4   5   6   7 Very easy

(5) How easy is it for the user to program the pump overall?

Very difficult 1   2   3   4   5   6   7 Very easy

Comments _____
_____
_____
_____

B. Use of instructional aids

(6) How often did the user refer to instructional aids? (Please circle one.)

Not at all   Occasionally   Often   Very often   Constantly

(7) Was the user able to resolve his/her issue(s) quickly? Yes _____ No _____

Comments _____
_____
_____
_____

IV. Summary comments, if any
_____
_____
_____
_____
_____
_____

Guiding Principles for Pump Implementation

Pamela K. Phelps

Key Terms

Alert fatigue—a tendency to ignore or minimize the potential negative impact of a technology alert, when presented with multiple alerts with varying degrees of importance.

DERS—dose error reduction software. In this case, it represents the programming of minimum and maximum dose limits in an infusion pump, and the alerts presented to the clinician when programmed doses are exceeded.

Drug library subset—a subset of the larger drug library that includes all drugs needed for a specific patient population or area. Other names that pump vendors use for these subsets are personalities, profiles, and clinical care areas.

Line labels—the practice of labeling infusion tubing in order to identify which medication is infusing in the tubing. For purposes of the smart pumps, the pump will display the drug name on the pump itself, perhaps obviating the need to label tubing lines.

Password protection—some pumps offer the added feature of requiring a password code to be input in order to gain access to a medication library, if the library is thought to include particularly high-risk medications, concentrations, or dose limits.

Scrolling—reading through drug names on the pump in order to find the desired drug name. If a drug list is fairly long, excessive scrolling can be inefficient.

The Need for Guiding Principles

On a vast project such as new pump implementation, it is wise for an oversight group to develop guiding principles. Guiding principles can be defined as a broad philosophy that guides an organization throughout its life in all circumstances, irrespective of changes in its goals, strategies, type of work, or the top management.[1] Principles are defined as fundamental norms, rules, or values that represent what is desirable and positive for a person, group, organization, or community, and help it in determining the rightfulness or wrongfulness of its actions.[1] By these definitions, guiding principles represent a general philosophy of what is right and wrong for the organization. A key point in the definition is that they do not change, regardless of changing circumstances around us. Using the guiding principles is helpful in making the tough decisions that may otherwise seem complex and fraught with controversy. Guiding principles should be developed by a group of individuals at a senior leadership level, such as chief nursing officers, pharmacy directors, and clinical nurse specialists.

Why are guiding principles needed in this process? Implementation groups will very quickly drill down from a macro level to a micro level. Each area of the hospital has a number of reasons why their processes exist as they are. And, each area of the hospital will advocate for their processes. Ideally, an institution will want to use pump implementation as a means of standardization of processes. If senior leadership sets out "standardization" as a guiding principle, this will challenge the implementation groups to look at new ways of achieving standardization.

Sample Guiding Principles

The following statements represent the use of guiding principles in decision-making regarding smart pump infusion technology. It is helpful to talk through these scenarios with your implementation team, prior to implementation.

Principle 1: Standardization of pump processes across the organization is our goal.[2,3]

Implication of this principle: When faced with differing opinions on pump deployment and in drug library decisions, this principle will help the group to come to consensus whenever possible.

Principle 2: Standardization of pumps is a means of obtaining efficiency and safety.[2,3]

Implication of this principle: Acknowledgement that non-standardization leads to inefficiency and potential medication errors. This will lead to a greater desire to standardize.

Principle 3: Medication pump programming for individual drug entities can vary throughout the organization.

Implication of this principle: Acknowledgement that maximum dosages and alerts will not be the same for a medication, dependent upon the placement of the patient (ICU, non-ICU). This principle balances the need for efficiencies in updating the pumps (programming one entry instead of several) with the individual needs of the nursing units (some units may use higher dosages of medications than others).[2,5] One compromise could be to apply an "80/20" rule to drug dosages. Create a standard that applies to the majority of situations, and create alternate processes for more unusual circumstances.

Principle 4: Area libraries will be standardized to the extent possible

Implication of this principle: This principle applies a common standard to any library location that has the same name. For example, each "med-surg" library will be standardized.[2] There is no single right answer to this principle. In fact, some sites advocate using separate locations or libraries for each care unit, in order to more precisely examine override reports.[4] Certainly, if varying dosage units are used (for example some units use mcg/min versus mcg/kg/min for blood pressure medication infusions), these varying units will need to be in separate locations to safely co-exist.

Principle 5: The primary purpose of the pump will be to avoid gross drug identification and drug calculation errors and support medication administration.

Implication of this principle: Dose limits will be designed to avoid gross errors in either identification or calculation. Your organization should ask, "How will we avoid a ten-times dosage error?" and "How can the pump aid in drug identification errors?," *not* "How can we use the pump to refine dosages for individual patients?" The pump process should support medication administration. A dose range setting in the pump that is too narrow may impede the provision of care to the patient. In addition, over-exposure to unnecessary alerts creates alert-fatigue and confusion regarding whether or not alerts are critical to patient safety.[5]

Principle 6: The pump will not be used as a means to *enforce* prescribing practices; rather it will be used to gauge adherence to policy and for policy refinement.

Implication of this principle: The purpose of the smart pump is to identify gross dosing errors; it cannot fix aberrant prescribing practices. As such, the DERS programming should not force the nurse to stop the delivery of care for dose refinement. Rather, dosages within the limits should be given. The report writing function should be used as a quality assurance tool to identify unusual prescribing practices, and to refine pump and drug policies.

Principle 7: Efforts should be made to avoid pump updates at a frequency greater than every 3 months.

Implication of this principle: The organization will need to decide what constitutes an emergency update, and what can wait until the next scheduled update. Updating the pump library and pushing the drug library is no small task, even if the system is wireless. Processes should be in place to handle regular updates, as well as urgent changes.[5]

Principle 8: Area libraries should be programmed such that a nurse in a given area should not be required to use more than one drug library, as a routine practice.

Implication of this principle: This principle is controversial, with no single right answer.[4] It requires careful discussion with the nursing leaders and pump users. Changing from one library location to another library location can be easy; however, it does require re-programming and some familiarity with the two separate locations. On the other hand, including an exhaustive list of medications that may be used in an area can lead to the need for excessive "scrolling" of the drug names in the library. Creating expectations is important; if a nurse expects that every drug is in the library, and cannot find the particular one they need, this can lead to frustration. It can also lead to the use of a generic entry such as "other drug." Use of a generic entry leads to use of the pump outside of any DERS programming, thereby negating any safety parameters.

Principle 9: Two care areas that share the same drug names, but use differing dose limits of dose expressions can be password-protected, with some pump brands.

Implications of this principle: Theoretically, all care areas will share common dose limits. However, if two sites both have anesthesia libraries, for example, and the physicians in those areas use different dose expressions (for example mcg/min versus mcg/kg/min), you may want to only allow access to these areas. Applying password technology (available on some pump models) can be difficult, depending upon the pump technology. If a password needs to be keyed into a pump, then each practitioner and nurse in the area will have to know the passcode.

Principle 10: Bolus doses should be programmed into the pump and given from an infusion bag whenever possible.[2, 7]

Implications of this principle: Certainly, not all bolus doses need to be given using an infusion pump. This principle refers to bolus doses that will be followed by a continuous infusion. Since newer smart pumps apply DERS technology to bolus doses as well as infusions, the general consensus is that it is safer to administer a bolus dose from an infusion bag.[2,7] It is important for the nurses and pharmacists to define how product will be sent from the pharmacy. Some pumps have a maximum infusion rate of 1000 mL/hr. So, if a heparin bolus is given from a heparin infusion bag, a bolus may take up to 6 minutes to infuse, depending upon the bag concentration. Nursing education regarding this change is important. Using a bolus infused call-back alarm feature may also be beneficial.

Principle 11: Using the pump to label infusion lines is a desirable safety measure, whether or not DERS technology is employed for a particular medication.

Implications of this principle: This principle would mean that line labels for a medication will display on the pump, even if no dose limits exist in the pump for that medication. This means that all medication names will be housed on the pump. Implications for nursing are that they will need to scroll through drug names to find the correct drug name. Some experts advocate limiting "line label only" medications in the drug library.[5] Some nurses may see this as inefficient; others may feel a measure of safety by having drug labels on the pump. Certainly you won't want to create time-wasters for nurses; there needs to be a payback for the practice. Your institution may decide that this practice is warranted because nurses label the medication lines already, to keep lines in order.[2] Medications that are labeled with a drug name on the pump will be easily identified by any care provider who is taking care of the patient, such as a new nurse coming on duty or a physician inspecting a patient's medications. In addition, reports generated by the pump software will be able to identify at what rates these medications are being run if there are any errors with them. It would be impossible to identify these errors if the lines were not labeled.

For Patient-Controlled Analgesia (PCA)

Principle 1: The PCA pump will be used in the following situations:

- For pain medication therapy with a patient-controlled activation order
- For general infusions of narcotics, for the purpose of securing Schedule II medications (unless other locking mechanisms are available)

Implication of this principle: This practice could be controversial. It says that general narcotic infusions will be given with a patient-controlled analgesia pump. This will be an institution specific decision. While it may ensure narcotic security, it also may be confusing to staff when using a PCA pump for a general infusion.

Principle 2: Concentrations of medications will be used that avoid frequent re-ordering of medication vials (>2 times/day).

Implication of this principle: The pharmacy will need to develop concentrations of medications that do not cause a need for excessive re-ordering of solutions. This may mean having multiple concentrations of narcotics or special compounding by the pharmacy.

Principle 3: High concentration narcotic infusions (with or without PCA) will be delivered using a large volume pump instead of the PCA pump.

Implications of this principle: Some institutions deliver high concentrations directly from a compounded fluid bag, instead of through a PCA pump. If your institution decides to provide high concentrations of narcotics via a large volume pump, separate checks and balances will need to be built in for these high-risk drugs.

Principle 4: The pharmacy will use commercially available (liquid) concentrations of drugs to prepare and dispense PCA medication.[2,7]

Implications of this principle: The organization should decide which commercially available products will be used. These can be obtained from a manufacturer, or outsourced to a compounding agency. Either way, the organization is responsible for the integrity of the product used. If this organization is USP-797 compliant[6] for Level 1 compounding, the organization could provide their own product, made from either liquids or powders.

Conclusion

Clearly, smart pump implementation is a complex process that will challenge your team to consider all current infusion practices for potential changes. It will be imperative for an implementation team to decide on guiding principles before pump implementation. Guiding principles can help us challenge the "status quo," and to obtain a new level of standardization of processes and policies. Along the way, individuals who have not been involved in the development of the guiding principles can be educated regarding the process and reasons for these principles. Guiding principles are a compass to help the implementation team and the organization guide their infusion pump decision-making.

PRACTICE TIPS

- Engage senior leaders to identify acceptable guiding principles for pump implementation; communicate guiding principles to those who are involved in the pump preparation and implementation.
- Re-evaluate guiding principles after pump implementation for validation.
- As the technology changes, more tools to enhance safety may become available. This may change the way the organization thinks about some of the principles. For example, it may become beneficial for care areas to become more unique, rather than more alike.

- Bring guiding principles to each pump meeting; chances are good that not all in attendance have been exposed to the principles, and will therefore bring different perspectives into the meeting.

References

1. businessdictionary.com. Accessed March 10, 2009.

2. Proceedings of a summit on preventing patient harm and death from I.V. medication errors. American Society of Health System Pharmacists. *Am J Health-Syst Pharm.* 2008;65:2367-2379.

3. Wilson K, Sullivan M. Preventing medication errors with smart infusion technology. *Am J Health-Syst Pharm.* 2004;61:177-183.

4. Siv-Lee L, Morgan L. Implementation of wireless "intelligent" pump IV infusion technology in a not-for-profit academic hospital setting. *Hosp Pharm.* 2007;42:832-840.

5. Breland BD, Michienzi KA. "Advancing patient safety with intelligent infusion technology." Paper presented at the American Society of Health-System Pharmacy Midyear Clinical Meeting, December 8, 2008.

6. U.S. Pharmacopeia. *USP <797> Guidebook to Pharmaceutical Compounding—Sterile Preparations.* Rockville, MD: U.S. Pharmacopeia; revised 2008.

7. Institute for Safe Medication Practices (ISMP). Proceedings from the ISMP Summit on the Use of Smart Infusion Pumps; Guidelines for Safe Implementation and Use.

Building a General Drug Library

Pamela K. Phelps and Michelle L. Borchart   **CHAPTER 5**

Key Terms

Bolus dose—a medication dose meant to be delivered over a very short period of time.[2]

Clinical care area—an area of the health system representing a certain group of patients who have similar patient care needs. For purposes of the infusion pump, a clinical care area is part of the pump programming that allows medications needed in the particular area to be separated into one particular list for one particular area. One example of a clinical care area is the intensive care unit.[2,3]

Dose rate units—units used to express the rate of infusion of a drug.

Drug library—a comprehensive list of medications and fluids that are to be delivered using the infusion pump. This library includes any dose, volume, or rate limitations that are programmed into the software.[2]

Drug library push—the act of updating pumps using wireless technology. The new drug library is "pushed" from the software housing the library out to the individual pumps.[2]

High "hard" dose limit—a high dose limit programmed into a pump; the pump cannot be programmed higher than a high "hard" limit. The user must use a dose lower than this limit.[2]

High "soft" dose limit—a high dose limit programmed into a pump; the pump will alert the user that the dose is unusually high, however, the user can still proceed with programming this dose.[2]

Infusion pump—a device that uses pressure to deliver specific volumes of fluid; used for fluid, blood and medication administration.

Low "hard" dose limit—a low dose limit programmed into a pump; the pump cannot be programmed lower than a low "hard" limit. The user must use a dose higher than this limit.[2]

Low "soft" dose limit—a low dose limit programmed into a pump; the pump will alert the user that the dose is unusually low, however, the user can still proceed with programming this dose.[2]

Nesting—grouping varying drug concentrations under a single drug name. This avoids having both concentrations show up on the main screen, thereby avoiding excessive scrolling.

Piggyback dose—a medication dose meant to be delivered over a relatively short period of time; this medication is infused through pump tubing that is connected to the primary infusion tubing.[2]

Smart infusion pumps—a new generation of infusion pumps that incorporates dose limiting software into the pump hardware; this software is designed to prevent infusion-related programming errors. The Joint Commission, in the 2006 National Patient Safety Goals, defined a smart pump as a "parenteral infusion pump equipped with IV medication error-prevention software that alerts operators or interrupts the infusion process when a pump setting is programmed outside of pre-configured limits. Smart pumps are designed to recognize prescription errors, dose misinterpretations, and keypad programming errors."[1]

Tall man lettering—a means of depicting drug names so that similar looking names can be differentiated. The part of the name that differentiates the two drugs is labeled with capital letters (for example, DOPamine, DOBUTamine).

Introduction

The building of a general large volume IV pump drug library starts with a pharmacist willing to build your facility drug library, a good IV medication reference, and the IV infusion pump that your facility is going to implement. It is important to have an actual pump available for the programmer during the building of the drug library in order to visualize what happens on the pump after limits are programmed into the computer. The programmer should learn how the pump works and play with the pump to get to know how it functions before starting to enter medications into the pump library. Medication limits entered into pump programming databases may cause unintended results when they are on the pump if the programmer does not regularly test programmed medication limits on the pump. This includes frequently "pushing" the drug library to the pump, in order to test the new functionality.

After the programmer has familiarized themselves with the pump and the programming software (or website), they are ready to start building the drug library.

Steps in Building the Library

Medication Name and Medication Display Name

Most smart pump software comes with a pre-defined list of medication names. This list will provide you with the basis of your pump library. For smaller hospitals, the vendor medication list will have most of the medication names that you need. For larger hospitals, this list may only contain 70% to 80% of the medications names needed for your library. Medication names can be added to the library list as needed (see Appendix A).

The next step is to choose the displayed name. The displayed name is what is displayed on the pump when the pump user chooses a medication. An important factor in the displayed name is "tall man" lettering for look-alike and sound-alike medications. For example the drug *dopamine* should be entered in as *DOPamine* to help differentiate it from other similarly spelled medications. This will help pump users differentiate between look-alike medications when searching for medications on the pump. The Hospira Symbiq, Sigma Spectrum, B Braun Outlook, and Alaris System all have screens with the ability to display tall man lettering.

If your institution or health system serves diverse patient populations such as adults, pediatrics, and neonates, it will be important for you to label medications as they correspond to your diverse patient populations. One option is to label pediatric medications as Drug-PEDS and to label neonatal medications as Drug-NICU. This naming convention allows for easy separation of the drug library to the appropriate drug library subsets later.[4] This method of naming medication also prevents programming errors. While inputting or editing limits of medications in the software, the programmer will be able to differentiate pediatric and neonatal medication entries from adult medication entries. This will avoid the error of entering wrong dosage limits; for example, entering adult medication dose limits into a pediatric medication entry could lead to an overdose error.

Medication Concentration

The next step in the programming process is entering the medication concentration. It is not required to enter a concentration for all medications. Many institutions and health systems may not have standard concentrations for their intravenous medications. These can still be entered into the pump programming, but each concentration will need to be entered as a separate medication. Some pumps allow nesting of medications with more than one concentration. *Nesting* is the term used when the user can select a medication name and the available concentrations immediately appear.[2] The advantage of nesting medications lies in the fact that the end user sees only the medication names on the pump screen while selecting a medication name for infusion. For example, if there are three concentrations of dopamine at the institution, they end user may have to see the name dopamine three times, one for each concentration. If the dopamine entry is nested, they see the name "dopamine" only once on the screen, select it, and the available concentrations immediately appear on the screen. This functionality is important to the end-user. It avoids extensive scrolling on the screen to find the correct medication name and concentration. Extensive scrolling and searching for medication names will greatly discourage buy-in from pump users.[5,6]

It is much easier to build limits for medications when concentrations are standardized, or limited to very few choices. In order to improve patient safety The Joint Commission included as one of the 2003 National Patient Safety Goals the requirement to "standardize and limit the number of drug concentrations available in the organization."[5,7,15] This highlights one of the advantages of implementing this technology. The health system will uncover variation in practice, and can take this opportunity to standardize.[5] This work can begin long before the pumps or software are available. Any time multiple "non-standard" concentrations are used for medications, an opportunity is introduced for user selection error.[5,7] In addition, added complexity and workload is created any time the pump library is modified and pushed, or updated and transferred wirelessly from a central server to the pumps.

Continuous Medication Dose Limits

Once a medication name, displayed name, and concentration (if applicable) have been entered, dosing rate units should be chosen for the dosing limits. Drug dose limits should be entered in the units in which the drug is most commonly prescribed. This will minimize the number of calculations that pump users will have to perform in programming medications for drug delivery.[5,8] Dosing rate units should also be chosen carefully. During this process, the programming pharmacist should perform frequent library pushes. What appears on the software can appear quite differently, once it is pushed to a pump. For example, anything dosed in units per day (such as mg/kg/day) may default to a 24-hour infusion on some pumps. You may run into situations where there is variability between clinicians in dosing units. For example, some practitioners use dosing units of mcg/min for vasopressors; others use mcg/kg/min. These differences in dosing units will require the programmer to enter these as separate medications. It is imperative that the bedside user choose the correct medication name for the dosing units prescribed. There are reports of medications being infused incorrectly by smart pump users due to having a different dosing rate unit in the pump than was ordered for a drug and causing serious errors.[5,8] Vasopressors are high-risk medications that carry a risk of catastrophic consequences if an error is made. If different dosing units are used in different care areas, these care areas should be separated into different libraries. Different dosing units in different care areas can be confusing for caregivers who work in both the care areas. We therefore encourage bedside caregivers to limit their work to one pump library as much as possible. This topic is discussed in greater depth in Chapter 9.

After dosing rate units are selected, dose limits can be entered. The choices for dosing limits include: low-hard limit, low-soft limit, high-soft limit, and high-hard limit. When a dose is entered that is above or below a soft limit, the pump will sound an alert, but the pump user will be able to override these limits. Soft limits inform the clinician that a dose is outside the recommended range, and require confirmation by the pump user that he or she intended to go beyond the usual dosage range.[2] If a dose is entered that is below a low hard limit or above a high hard limit, a pump user will not be able to override this limit. He or she will only have the option of editing the medication dose, in order to infuse that medication on the pump. Therefore, it is important to set hard limits wide enough so that your users will be able to administer any dose needed for a particular medication. If the hard limits are too narrow, the pump will not allow that dose to be given without the user selecting the "other drug" function. Use of "other drug" as a medication selection is discouraged because it requires the user to operate the pump outside of the programmed safety limits. Hard limits may be set differently for different areas; for example, the institution may want to set broader limits for the intensive care unit, the operating room, and the emergency department. There is a fine balance in setting hard limits; the health system will want hard limits that prevent catastrophic overdoses. Most institutions will set broad hard limits while first implementing a new pump. Over time, these hard limits can be fine-tuned and perhaps narrowed to meet the needs of the patient population safely.[3]

There is some flexibility in choosing whether or not to assign dose limits to medications in the library. For example, low limits are intended to prevent under-dosing of medications. They generally are not needed for maintenance IV fluids. They also may pose nuisance alerts for medications that are frequently tapered when discontinued, such as vasopressors.[9] Lower limits may be more important for medications where under-dosing leads to an undesirable effect, such as chemotherapy or narcotic analgesics. The health system should carefully consider whether or not to use low limits, and when these low limits should be assigned. Note that not all pumps have the ability to assign low limits.

If your institution is converting from an older style pump to a new pump, it will be beneficial to start with the medications and dosage limits database from your previous pump as a starting point. If you are not converting from a pump with a dose-limiting database, start with your institution's formulary of intravenous medications and a list of the most commonly used intravenous medications. When entering medications into the pump database, the software will generally place the medications in alphabetical order. It is important to include all intravenous medications that may be used in your health system.[8] This inclusiveness will minimize the number of infusions run outside of the drug library limits under "other drug." "Other drug" should only be used when a medication name is not included in the drug library, since using "other drug" is working outside of the dose checking parameters of the pump. Hospitals with an active investigational drug area will need to consider adding an investigational drug library.

When programming medications into the pump, it is recommended to have a single pharmacist working in the database. Allowing only one pharmacist access to programming will reduce confusion or mix-ups that will occur with multiple programmers. When entering medications into the database, use the medication tables at the end of this chapter, as well as standard drug references. Decide which medications are candidates for high limits and low limits. Once all of the medications are entered into the library, the limits should be reviewed by a group of healthcare practitioners for feedback. Continuous medication dose limits are listed in Appendix A. *Disclaimer: This information is provided for demonstration purposes only. ASHP makes no representations about the validity, accuracy, reliability or suitability of the information, specifically disclaims liability for consequences that may arise in connection with the information, and urges practitioners to exercise their best professional judgments about the dosing limits presented. Dosing limits should be based upon hospital utilization patterns, as well as on acceptable dosing ranges. Practitioners are advised that some of the dosing limits presented here may exceed FDA-approved doses. This was done to avoid excessive alerts and alert fatigue. Practitioners are advised to use caution when determining appropriate dosing limits.*

Special Considerations: Antimicrobials, IV Fluids, Blood Products

Certain medications may be easier to enter as generic line items, instead of listing out each medication separately. An example of this includes most antimicrobial agents. Most antimicrobial agents can be infused over a time period of 30 to 60 minutes, and are relatively low-risk for side effects. If each antimicrobial agent were listed separately in the drug library, the medication list would become very large and cumbersome. Lengthening the list of medications in the library will lengthen the time the user spends in searching for the correct medication name. This can be a user dissatisfier. To avoid this inconvenience, the health system can list antimicrobials in the drug library by volume. For example, antibiotics can be listed as antibiotic 50 mL, antibiotic 100 mL, antibiotic 150 mL, antibiotic 250 mL, etc. Then limits can be set on the antibiotics in mL/hr so that the antibiotics would be run over approximately 30–60 minutes. Exceptions to listing antimicrobials in this manner include vancomycin and amphotericin B. These agents can cause infusion reactions if run too quickly. It is recommended to list these agents independently with specific limits. It may also be beneficial to list aminoglycosides separately, in order to ensure they are run over a specific amount of time. This will aid in accurate pharmacokinetic calculations and drug dosing. Despite any inconvenience, some institutions elect to add all antimicrobial agent names individually to the drug library.

Other items that would be cumbersome to list out individually are IV fluids. IV fluids are generally safe and low risk if infused too quickly. Our recommendation for adults is to have one entry for general IV fluids with limits and to have a separate entry for IV fluids with potassium with much tighter limits. Separate entries will be required for IV fluids and IV fluids with potassium for pediatrics and neonates. Blood products may also be listed as one line item with broad limits or no limits. Infusion practices for blood products is highly varied; often it is essential to run blood fairly quickly, hence the need for very broad limits.

If your health system does not have a chemotherapy library or is still in the development stages of the chemotherapy library, it is a good idea to have a chemotherapy line item with no limits. If a chemotherapy line item is entered in the pump, then at the nurse will have a label visible on the pump and know the agent infusing is chemotherapy. This will also allow anyone else caring for the patient to be able to easily see that the medication infusing on the pump is chemotherapy. It will also give the pump user an item to select when programming chemotherapy for infusion.

If you include additional medications in your drug library or choose to build your limits independently, it is important to use one or more quality drug references to aid in building drug limits. We recommend *Intravenous Medications: A Handbook for Nurses and Health Professionals*, Gahart and Nazareno (Mosby)[10] and *Pediatric Injectable Drugs*, 9th edition ("The Teddy Bear Book," American Society of Health-System Pharmacists).[13]

Bolus Doses

Whenever possible, the smart pump should be used to infuse bolus doses of intravenous medications. Delivering bolus doses via the smart pump improves safety and avoids human error in drug administration. This is accomplished by programming dosing limits for boluses in the pump software. There are some situations where it is not feasible to administer the bolus dose using the smart pump. These situations are generally those in which the concentration of the maintenance infusion is such that the volume of the bolus dose would be either too large or too small to administer safely with the smart pump. In these situations it may be better to either hang a separate bag on the smart pump as a bolus dose or administer the bolus dose push with a syringe.

The pump programmer must enter each medication that should be enabled to be delivered as a bolus or loading dose, along with the continuous infusions.[7,8] Medications that will be given as a bolus using the pump should have the "bolus" feature enabled during programming. Dose limits should be identified for those medications with the bolus feature enabled.

Bolus limits can be entered in two different ways; they can be entered as amounts (mg, g, etc.) or rates. If bolus limits are entered as amounts, time limits can be programmed for the bolus so that it will not be administered too fast or too slow. Bolus rate limits are in the same units as continuous rate limits, and will limit the rate of a bolus. As with continuous rate limits, there are lower hard limits, lower soft limits, upper soft limits, and upper hard limits. Again it is the institution's choice to enter all, none, or some of the limits, for all, none, or some of the medications. These decisions should be made based on the patient-care needs, balanced against the risk for adverse events and the potential toxicity of the medication. Bolus dose limits are included in Appendix A.

Delivery Methods

The next programming function is to determine the delivery methods available for each medication. The available delivery methods include basic, piggyback, intermittent, and multistep. The basic or continuous infusion is the default mode that most infusions will utilize. A piggyback infusion allows the infuser to deliver fluid from a secondary container at a rate and volume independent of the primary infusion.[2] A piggyback is also referred to as a secondary infusion. An intermittent therapy delivers at regular intervals in "on and off" cycles for the entire therapy (for example, to give a medication every 4 hours).[2]

A multistep therapy is used for medications such as parenteral nutrition that begin at a starting rate for a period of time, then increase to a new rate.[2] The multistep option may also be referred to as a "ramp up" or "taper" option. This feature may not be present in every brand of pump. Each medication in the pump drug library should be evaluated for the potential to be infused using the various delivery methods; basic, piggyback, intermittent, and multistep. Do not use the intermittent delivery method for medications where interruption of the infusion will result in untoward patient outcomes, such as vasopressors.

Delivery at End of Infusion

Another important part of programming each medication is selection of the delivery at end of infusion. This is what occurs after the volume to be infused (VTBI) programmed by the pump user has finished, and before the next bag is hung. In most pumps the only option for delivery at end of infusion is KVO (Keep Vein Open), but the KVO can be set at varying rates. Rates generally range from 0–20 mL/hr in the majority of pumps or up to 50 mL/hr in the Sigma Spectrum. The default KVO rate will be set by the institution. This rate can be different for each medication. It can also be set differently for pediatric medications and adult medications according to patient care needs. In most circumstances the KVO rate can be changed by the pump user for each medication when programming the pump.

Some pumps have expanded programming options for delivery at end of infusion including: None, Continuous and KVO. Choosing "None" will stop the infusion and no additional fluid will be delivered. This may be a good choice for chemotherapy medications where no additional medication should be delivered beyond the specified volume. "Continuous" should be chosen to continue to deliver the programmed rate at the end of the infusion. "Continuous" would be used for medications such as pressor agents where a change in medication rate could lead to a patient's clinical deterioration. The "KVO" option will change to a rate set by the institution, typically in a range of 0.1–20 mL/hr.[2] This setting would be used for medications such as IV fluids, which are commonly used to keep veins open.

The delivery at end of infusion section requires extensive nursing collaboration. Nurses will need to determine which medications should have:

- no delivery at the end of infusion of the VTBI
- delivery at a continuous rate at the end of infusion of the VTBI
- default to KVO at the end of the infusion of the VTBI

Nurses will also determine the KVO rate for adult and pediatric medications.

Enable Stand-By and Piggyback

An option for programming that delays the beginning of infusions of medications is the "enable stand-by" feature. This is also termed a "delay infusion" feature. If stand-by programming is enabled, this allows the infusion to begin at a later time than when the pump was programmed, and to be switched on and off during the infusion.[2] The "enable stand-by" feature is commonly used in areas such as the operating room, where patient care infusion needs may be anticipated prior to surgery. It may also be used in the intensive care unit when anticipating critical transfers from other hospitals, when it is known that the patient is receiving vital infusion medications.

Another programming feature is the "enable piggyback and bolus from secondary when medication is infusing." If this feature is chosen, it will allow the primary infusion to be interrupted to administer a piggyback or bolus from a secondary container, while the primary medication is infusing.[2] This feature should be disabled for medications that cannot be interrupted, such as vasopressors, narcotics, and sedatives. Nursing collaboration will be required to determine which medications can be interrupted to administer a piggyback. This feature is not available on all pump brands.

See Appendix A for a list of recommendations for specific delivery methods, high-risk medications, delivery at end of infusion, enabling stand-by, and enabling piggybacks.

Clinical Notes

Many of the newer smart pumps allow for the ability to enter customized clinical notes or messages to the pump user. These messages can be built to be drug-specific. Clinical notes will then appear whenever the drug in question is selected. The notes can provide the user safety and medication administration information such as "filter required" or "central line only." We advise judicious use of clinical notes. Too many clinical notes may give the pump user alert fatigue, resulting in the user bypassing important clinical information. The health system may choose to program clinical notes only for medications where errors are common or risk of error is significant.

Vendor Support

Vendor support can be obtained when building a drug library. The vendor role in the drug library build is generally limited to training the pharmacists to use the pump software. The vendor will also explain the consequences of the various programming specifications that will be built into the pump software. Vendor representatives will help with basic pump specification decisions such as alarm settings and occlusion pressure settings. Vendors will offer examples of what other institutions have done, but will generally advise customizing the settings to your health system.

Most vendors will not offer specific advice regarding dose limits due to liability concerns. They also stress customization of the drug library to meet the needs of the hospital or health system patient population.

Vendors will be present during pump go-live. The amount of vendor support for go-live is determined during contracting. Vendors will train super-users and provide support during the "switch-out" of old pumps for new models.

Nursing Collaboration

When building the pump drug library, nursing involvement in the process is essential. Nurses will be the end users of the pump; as such, they will want input into what is in the drug library, the drug limits, the various settings on each medication, and in what order they appear in the drug library. Since nurses will be the ones using the pump, they should be involved in the smart pump process from the beginning. A committee will oversee the multidisciplinary process, including nursing, pharmacy and other health care providers, engaging nurses to help with the building and refining of the drug library.

Review of Drug Library Limits

Once limits have been established and all other settings have been entered for the drug library, it is good practice to have the limits reviewed by a group of practitioners from different practice areas. Pharmacists should review the limits for adherence to drug policy and dosage limits. Nurses will address the processes of how medications are administered in everyday practice. Nurses will also need to determine various pump settings, such as delivery at end of infusion for each medication.

Conclusion

Programming intelligent infusion pumps is a multiple step process. Understanding how the medication specifications "look" on the pump is crucial to the development of a usable pump library. While some of these specifications can be taken from standard infusion references, others require collaboration with nurses and other healthcare professionals. It is imperative to seek multi-disciplinary feedback for this process. The pump programming should begin with existing nursing policy and practice regarding delivering medication, fluid, and blood infusions. Some specifications will require that a health system take a careful look at infusion policies and practices that need to be incorporated into the pump programming. Variations in infusion practices will be brought to light during this discovery process. The goal of this examination of infusion policies should be to standardize practices regarding drug concentrations, high-risk drugs, and drug delivery methods.

PRACTICE TIPS

- Think of the main drug library as you think of a library for an mp3 player. Your mp3 player has a general library that includes all the songs you own. You can then allocate each of these songs to a playlist. Songs can be in multiple playlists. In this analogy, the songs in the general library represent medication names, and their associated dose limits. The playlist represents care areas where the medication names will appear.
- For medications such as maintenance fluids or TPN, where a concentration will not be entered into the pump, it is important to check the "no concentration" button when programming. This will avoid an unnecessary prompt to pump users to enter a medication concentration while programming an infusion.
- Establish a multidisciplinary team. Make sure existing infusion policies and practices are known to the team prior to programming the pump.[7]
- It is imperative that there is a nursing representative from each area of the hospital where the pump will be implemented. This allows for a voice from the end user. Clearly needs may be different in the ICU as compared to outpatient infusion, for example. Nurses also need to acknowledge and prepare to train for any changes in existing infusion processes that are brought about with the new pump.
- Make sure you have a pump in hand before programming. Push a library to a pump early (and often) in the process, so that you can identify any special considerations in how the drug displays on the pump.
- Decide on drug naming conventions <u>before</u> starting to program the pump.
- Consider what you would like to use for a display name. For example, if you are programming separate limits for PEDS, NICU, and ADULT, consider a display name of "DOPamine PEDS," "DOPamine NICU," or "DOPamine ADULT" to make sorting into care areas easier.
- Order sets and pathways should be considered prior to programming the pump limits.

- Identify any investigational protocols that use extraordinary doses of medications. Consider having a special nomenclature built into the pump for these medications.
- If you already have pump libraries from an older version pump, use this as your basis for going forward.
- It may be easier to enter all your medications, continuous dose limits and bolus limits into the drug library first and then later go back through and edit the rest of the features.
- Beginning the process of standardizing medication concentrations prior to pump software programming will save a lot of time in the long run. For each medication, try to limit the number of different concentrations. Too many concentrations for an infusion medication will lead to confusion and error.
- Decide which medications nurses will be administering by bolus or piggyback. Inherent in this decision is judging which medication infusions can be interrupted to administer a piggyback infusion.
- Standardize practice for delivery at end of infusion.

References

1. ERCI Institute. General Purpose Infusion Pumps. *Health Devices.* 2007;36:309-339.

2. Hospira Corporation. Hospira MedNet® Meds User Guide. Version 5.1. September 2007.

3. Siv-Lee L, Morgan L. Implementation of wireless "intelligent" pump IV infusion technology in a not-for-profit academic hospital setting. *Hosp Pharm.* 2007;42:832-840.

4. Breland B, Michienzi K. Advancing patient safety with intelligent infusion technology. Paper presented at: American Society of Health System Pharmacy Midyear Meeting; Orlando, FL; 2008.

5. Pennsylvania Patient Safety Authority. Smart infusion pump technology: don't bypass the safety catches. *Patient Saf Advis.* 2007;4:1-6.

6. McAlearney AS, Vrontos J, Schneider PJ. Strategic Work-arounds to accommodate new technology: the case of smart pumps in hospital care. *J Patient Saf.* 2007;3:75-81.

7. Institute for Safe Medication Practices. Effective Approaches to Standardization and Implementation of Smart Pump Technology. (www.ismp.org/smartpumpce/default.asp) Accessed January 2009.

8. Bates DW, Vanderveen T, Seger D, et al. Variability in Intravenous Medication Practices: Implications for Medication Safety. *Jt Comm J Qual Patient Saf.* 2005;31:203-210.

9. Institute for Safe Medication Practices. Effective Approaches to Standardization and Implementation of Smart Pump Technology. (www.ismp.org/smartpumpce/default.asp) Accessed January 2009.

10. Gahart DB, Nazareno AR. *Intravenous Medications A Handbook for Nurses and Health Professionals.* 26th ed. St. Louis, MO: Mosby Elsevier; 2010.

11. Trissel LA. *Handbook on Injectable Drugs.* 15th ed. Bethesda, MD: American Society of Health-System Pharmacists; 2008.

12. Lacy CF, Armstrong LL, Goldman MP, Lance LL. Lexi-Comp's *Drug Information Handbook.* 17th ed. Hudson, NY: Lexi-Comp; 2008.

13. Phelps SJ, Hak EB, Crill CM. *The Teddy Bear Book: Pediatric Injectable Drugs.* 9th ed. Bethesda, MD: American Society of Health-System Pharmacists; 2010.

14. Micromedex DRUGDEX® System [Internet database]. Greenwood Village, CO: Thomson Reuters (Healthcare) Inc. Updated periodically.

15. Rich DS. Ask the Joint Commission: more on the requirements of the medication-related national patient safety goals for 2003–2004. *Hosp Pharm.* 2003;38:977-980.

16. American Hospital Formulary Service Drug Information 2009. American Society of Health System Pharmacists. Bethesda, MD.

Drug Library Development for Patient Controlled Analgesia

Virginia L. Ghafoor

Key Terms

Common PCA Administration Terminology[1,2]

Continuous infusion (basal rate, background infusion)—an analgesic medication administered at a constant rate (mg/hr or mcg/hr).

Demand dose (PCA dose, incremental dose)—quantity of an analgesic medication administered by the patient upon activation of the dose button linked to the PCA pump.

Dose limit—total amount of an analgesic medication that can be given in any 1- or 4-hour period.

Dose variables—drug selection, initial loading dose, PCA dose, lockout interval, infusion rate, dose limits.

Loading dose (bolus dose)—clinician (nurse or physician) activated dose administered through the PCA pump for initial titration to the MEAC.

Minimum effective analgesic concentration (MEAC)—the lowest steady-state serum concentration of an analgesic medication at which pain is relieved.

Mode of administration (delivery mode)—PCA dose only, continuous infusion only, PCA dose plus continuous infusion.

Patient controlled analgesia (PCA)—a conceptual framework for administration of analgesics to provide immediate delivery of the medication upon patient demand. PCA is not restricted to a single class of analgesics, routes, or modes of administration (for example: IV, PCA; epidural, PCEA).

Time interval (lockout)—minimum allowable period between patient-activated PCA doses.

Drug Library Program Terminology (from Chapter 5)

High "soft" dose limit (HSL)—a high dose limit programmed into a pump; the pump will alert the user that the dose is unusually high, however, the user can still proceed with programming this dose.

High "hard" dose limit (HHL)—a high dose limit programmed into a pump; the pump cannot be programmed higher than a high "hard" limit. The user must use a dose lower than this limit.

Low "soft" dose limit (LSL)—a low dose limit programmed into a pump; the pump will alert the user that the dose is unusually low, however, the user can still proceed with programming this dose.

Low "hard" dose limit (LHL)—a low dose limit programmed into a pump; the pump cannot be programmed lower than a low "hard" limit. The user must use a dose higher than this limit.

Introduction

The scope of discussion for PCA drug library development in this chapter will focus on intravenous (IV) medications. A PCA drug library contains information that is used to program the pump for delivery mode and dose variables. The Institute for Safe Medication Practices (ISMP) recommends use of smart PCA pumps with dose error reduction software (DERS) that alarms when problems are detected with programming of dose variables. Lower and upper limits for detection of errors are important safety functions built into the PCA drug library.[3] These limits vary depending on the clinical care area, nursing practice, and institution policies for medication use. Therefore, development of the PCA drug library is a multidisciplinary effort.

The multidisciplinary team should include clinical nursing and pharmacy staff responsible for care of adult and pediatric patients, technology support personnel, and education specialists from each hospital in the healthcare organization. It has been suggested that the team leader be a manager whose role involves integration of clinical practice and patient safety throughout the healthcare organization.[4] This enables the healthcare organization to develop a centralized process to support and maintain the PCA drug library. The steps involved in developing the PCA drug library are discussed in the next section.

Drug Library Development for PCA Pumps

Clinical Practice Guidelines

The drug library may be specific to a practice setting or patient population for delivery mode and/or dose variable limits. Integration of the PCA pump with clinical care involves consideration of several factors including evidence-based pain management guidelines, medication safety recommendations, institutional practice pertaining to analgesic use and PCA standard order sets (see Table 6-1).

Key objectives for drug library development should focus on:

- Use of drug library names that are easily identified.
- Avoiding creation of multiple libraries with duplication of information.
- Coordination with standard PCA orders sets.
- Compliance with institutional policies (refer to Table 6-2 for examples).

Table 6-1. Integration of Clinical Practice and PCA

Clinical Practice	Factors to Consider for PCA Integration
Opioid naive patients	• Does your institution have opioid dose limits to minimize unintended respiratory depression in naïve patients? • Is the delivery mode restricted to loading dose and PCA dose functions? • Does your institution use a standard PCA order set specific for opioid naive patients?
Opioid tolerant patients	• Does your institution have limits on opioid dose titration for tolerant patients? • Are multiple delivery modes used (i.e., loading dose, continuous infusion and PCA dose)? • Does your institution use a standard PCA order set specific for opioid tolerant patients?
Postoperative	• Is the delivery mode restricted to loading dose and PCA dose functions in the PACU? • Do surgical order sets containing analgesic medications address the PCA delivery mode?
Intensive care (ICU)	• Is the PCA pump being used for continuous infusion with no patient activated dosing (i.e., pump not being used under the intent of PCA)? • Does the opioid dose used sedation and analgesia require higher dose limits (i.e., fentanyl)? • Does the ICU practice setting have limits on opioid titration? • Do order sets addressing analgesic medication specify delivery mode for PCA pumps?
High concentration/ high dose	• Does your institution have patient populations using large doses of opioids (i.e., palliative care, oncology) • Are multiple delivery modes used (i.e., continuous infusion and PCA dose)? • Does your institution have patients with extremely high opioid requirements that exceed the infusion capacity of the pump with standard opioid concentrations?
Nonstandard analgesics	• Does your institution treat patients with intractable pain that is refractory to standard opioids (i.e., methadone infusion used for refractory pain). • Are analgesic medications other than pure mu opioid agonists administered through PCA (i.e., nalbuphine, ketamine).

The drug library name should be a term that is common to staff. Limit number of characters in the name to fit the size of the visual display screen on the pump (maximum character limits vary depending on manufacturer). Use of "tallman" lettering for look-alike and sound-alike medications (e.g., HYDROmorphone) can improve safety with name recognition between morphine and hydromorphone. Eliminate the use of similar libraries that may lead to programming errors due to incorrect selection.[5]

It is important that each drug library be coordinated with PCA standard orders. The PCA order set serves as a guide for drug selection, dosing and time interval. The ISMP recommends that healthcare organizations require the use of standard PCA order sets.[5] As an example, separate drug libraries should be created so standard PCA order sets for opioid naive and opioid tolerant patients will correlate to the appropriate delivery mode and dose variable limits.[6] For pediatric patients, weight-based CCAs should be used for opioid naive and opioid tolerant PCA order sets (refer to Chapter 7, on the pediatric drug library). The use of a flow diagram is helpful in teaching staff the relationship between the PCA order set and drug library selection.

Many healthcare institutions have policies pertaining to clinical setting, nursing practice, pharmacy distribution, and restrictions for use of PCA medications (refer to Table 6-2). Some policies may be specific to opioids that create limits for the drug library (i.e., restrictions on meperidine, opioid range orders). The policies may need to be updated prior to implementing new PCA pump technology to reflect new clinical practice changes.

Medication and Dose Parameters

Drug Selection

The choice of opioid for PCA is guided by clinical practice protocols and patient medical history. Analgesic effects of opioids are mainly a result of opioid mu-receptor binding. Morphine, hydromorphone and fentanyl are pure opioid mu-receptor agonists commonly used for PCA administration. Morphine is considered the prototype for opioid administration via PCA based on numerous well-designed clinical studies found in literature.[2,7,8] The peak effect (equilibration time between the blood and brain) after IV morphine administration is about 15–30 minutes. Plasma morphine concentrations after rapid IV injection do not correlate closely with the pharmacologic effect presumably due to the delay in penetration across the blood-brain barrier (i.e., morphine is water soluble). As a result, the analgesic and ventilatory depressant effects of IV morphine may not be evident with initial high plasma concentrations.[9]

Hydromorphone is commonly used in patients who cannot tolerate morphine or have a history of renal insufficiency. Hydromorphone is a hydrogenated ketone analogue of morphine with slightly higher lipid solubility. The peak effect after IV hydromorphone administration is between 8–20 minutes.[10,11]

Table 6-2. Example of Policies Impacting PCA Use

Nursing Practice

Purpose: Provide nursing staff with a guide to assist in the evaluation, treatment, and monitoring of the patient with PCA.

Policy:

- For the patient's safety, no one but the patient administers PCA (intermittent boluses) medication.
- PCA is only appropriate for patients who are capable of understanding self-dosing, who are capable of manipulating the dosing button, and whose visitors refrain from pushing the button. If these criteria cannot be met, then the PCA option must be deleted and nurse-administered dosing must be substituted.
- The pump may be used for opioid infusions without the PCA function in order to secure controlled substances.

Post Anesthesia Care Unit (PACU)

Purpose: Patient-controlled analgesia is a method by which patients can administer small doses of narcotic via a pump connected to their IV line. This method allows patients to control their own therapy. Initiating PCAs in the PACU at discharge helps patients maintain adequate comfort levels as they are transported from the PACU to their patient care units.

Policy:

- Patients considered for the PCA mode of administration must be able to understand and comply with instructions.
- No one but the patient administers PCA medications.
- Clinician–activated boluses are NOT be used in PACU.
- PCA pumps are programmed according to surgeon's post-op orders.
- The PCA pump is placed in line for patient to use only as needed on return to the PCU. Exception: Patients on continuous infusion rates both pre- and intra-operatively may remain on the continuous rate in PACU.

High Risk Medication

Purpose: To provide for the safety of procurement, storage, and preparation and distribution of high risk medications.

Policy:

PCA Procedure

- Includes manufactured products and those batch compounded by a compounding pharmacy.
- Must be prescribed on a specified PCA order form approved by a pharmacy and therapeutics committee.
- Must be infused on the smart PCA pump.
- Includes: morphine 25 mg/mL, hydromorphone 10 mg/mL, methadone10 mg/mL, nalbuphine 10 mg/mL and standard concentrations compounded patient specific.
- May not be available on override from the Pyxis cabinet.
- When stored in the Pyxis cabinet, these products must be stored in non-matrix (individual) compartments.

Continued

Table 6-2. Example of Policies Impacting PCA Use (cont'd)

Narcotic Range Order

Purpose: This policy provides guidelines for ordering opioid medications. The intent is to establish limits for safe opioid administration.

Policy:
- Range orders can be utilized when opioid dosing fluctuates frequently based on the patient's pain control.
- The highest dose in a range should not exceed two times the lowest dose in the range. For example, if a range order for morphine is written with a starting dose of 1 mg, it will read "morphine 1–2 mg."
- This policy applies to all dosage forms of narcotics, including patient-controlled analgesia orders (PCA), bolus doses, infusion doses, intra-muscular doses, oral doses, subcutaneous doses, rectal doses, and transmucosal doses.

Meperidine

Purpose: To limit meperidine (Demerol®) use to safe and appropriate applications in order to avoid drug toxicity.

Policy:

Temporary use of meperidine will be limited to prevention of rigors, post-anesthesia shivering and acute pain situations not exceeding a maximum of 600 mg IV per 24 hours and duration of use beyond 48 hours.

Meperidine should not be used in the following situations:
- Long-term pain management
- Patients with renal insufficiency (with the exception of pre-meds)
- Patients taking mono-amine oxidase inhibitors (MAO inhibitors)
- Intravenous patient controlled analgesia (PCA)

Source: Excerpts are from policies at the University of Minnesota Medical Center, Fairview.

Fentanyl is a synthetic phenylpiperidine compound with high lipid solubility resulting in rapid transfer across the blood-brain barrier. The peak effect after IV fentanyl administration can be seen within 5–6 minutes.[9,12] Fentanyl is a good option for patients who are allergic to morphine or have renal impairment.[13]

Meperidine is no longer recommended for use in PCA due to the risk of neurotoxicity with normeperidine metabolite accumulation.[2,7] The data on non-standard medications for PCA use such as methadone, sufentanil, ketamine, and nalbuphine is limited to small studies and case reports.[2,8,14-16] PCA drug library development for non-standard medications requires a review of literature for evidence-based efficacy and safety. Non-standard medications with a high risk for adverse events should have restrictions on personnel authorized for prescribing and administration. There are some PCA pump models available that have password protection to restrict unauthorized personnel from administering medications that are non-standard, high-risk and/or investigational. Non-standard medications administered via the PCA pump but not on standard order sets due to unique practice limitations should be in a separate drug library.

Concentration

The central issue with drug concentration is patient safety. Dosing errors due to inadvertently programming a *lower* than actual concentration of opioid into the PCA pump results in a *higher* PCA dose than prescribed. This can result in serious respiratory depression and death. Opioids and sedatives are considered high-risk medications for serious adverse events by ISMP. ISMP recommendations for limiting opioid concentrations include[3]:

- Use a single concentration for each drug when possible
- Use of custom concentrations should be restricted to selected patient care areas
  - Example: low concentration for small opioid doses used by neonates
  - Example: high concentration for large opioid doses used by patients with high opioid tolerance
- Use a distinct label for custom concentrations that is different in color and appearance from standard PCA labeling

In July 2008, a multidisciplinary summit meeting was convened to discuss goals for preventing patient harm and death from IV medication errors. With respect to drug concentrations, workgroup participants proposed actions for regulatory and statutory agencies to[17]:

- Require nationally standardized infusion concentrations for medication most frequently associated with harm or death
- Require standardized and distinct concentrations for IV, epidural and intrathecal administration devices
- Request expedited process for Food and Drug Administration approval of additional infusion concentration for currently approved drugs

It is recommended that healthcare institutions have a high-risk medication policy (refer to Table 6-2) that restricts the use of concentrated opioid infusions to smart PCA pumps with DERS technology.[3,17]

Loading Dose

Use of a loading dose accelerates the effective blood levels of the opioid at the initiation of therapy.[18] The initial loading dose allows for titration of medication when activated by the programmer (not the patient). The initial loading dose can be used by nurses in the postanesthesia care unit (PACU) to titrate opioid to the MEAC or by post surgical and medical nurses for "breakthrough" bolus doses.[2] Common equivalent IV loading doses for starting therapy in adults are morphine 2 mg, hydromorphone 0.3 mg, or fentanyl 20 mcg.[2] Opioids with long half-lives (i.e., methadone and levorphanol) should not be used for rapid titration because the duration of action may outlast declining pain stimuli, increasing the risk of opioid-induced adverse side effects including respiratory depression.[7]

Since there is marked interpatient variability in the MEAC, the loading dose needs to be administered in individualized and appropriate increments. The loading dose should be repeated three times if the patient's pain is not relieved rapidly.[17] If nurse-administered dosing is ordered via the PCA pump, the upper hard limit should not exceed a total beyond three doses for opioid naive patients (refer to Table 6-3a). If an opioid naive patient requires more than three nurse-administered loading doses for two or more consecutive hours, an evaluation is needed to assess the patient's opioid tolerance and ability to use the demand dose button for further adjustments to the PCA regimen.[2,18] Opioid tolerant patients will require larger loading doses and higher upper dose limits (refer to Table 6-3b).

The lower drug limit feature on some PCA pump models is not particularly useful for loading doses since a finite number of doses are given per protocol. In most cases, the lower limit should be fixed at the minimum amount of drug that can be infused by the pump.

PCA Dose

There is no established superior dosing regimen for IV PCA demand dose and lockout interval.[2] The hourly limit on the PCA pump should be set to three to five times the projected hourly requirement.[7] The ranges of usual maintenance doses for hydromorphone, morphine, and fentanyl are found in Table 6-4.[2]

For opioid naive patients, standard drug concentrations should be used to prevent unintentional overdosing. The lower pump limits are fixed at the minimum amount of drug that can be infused by the pump at the specified concentration. The initial upper dose limit for opioid naive patients should be more conserva-

Table 6-3(a). Example of Dose Limits for Adult Opioid Naive Patients

Drug	Parameter	Lower Soft Limit	Lower Hard Limit	Upper Soft Limit	Upper Hard Limit
Hydromorphone 1 mg/mL	Loading dose	0.1 mg	0.1 mg	0.3 mg	1 mg
	PCA dose	0.1 mg	0.1 mg	0.2 mg	0.4 mg
	Continuous	None; not permitted on standard orders			
	Dose limit	None	None	2.4 mg	3.6 mg
	Time interval	1-hour period			
Morphine 1 mg/mL	Loading dose	0.1 mg	0.1 mg	2 mg	6 mg
	PCA dose	0.1 mg	0.1 mg	1 mg	3 mg
	Continuous	None; not permitted on standard orders			
	Dose limit	None	None	12 mg	18 mg
	Time interval	1-hour period			
Fentanyl 50 mcg/mL	Loading dose	5 mcg	5 mcg	25 mcg	75 mcg
	PCA dose	5 mcg	5 mcg	25 mcg	40 mcg
	Continuous	None; not permitted on standard orders			
	Dose limit	None	None	200 mcg	300 mcg
	Time Interval	1-hour period			

Source: Fairview Health Services, Hospira Lifecare PCA Pump Drug Library.

Table 6-3(b). Example of Dose Limits for Adult Opioid Tolerant Patients

Drug	Parameter	Lower Soft Limit	Lower Hard Limit	Upper Soft Limit	Upper Hard Limit
Hydromorphone 1 mg/mL	Loading dose	0.1 mg	0.1 mg	1 mg	10 mg
	PCA dose	0.1 mg	0.1 mg	2 mg	5 mg
	Continuous	0.1 mg/hr	0.1 mg/hr	10 mg/hr	20 mg/hr
	Dose limit	None	None	20 mg	20 mg
	Time interval	1-hour period			
Morphine 5 mg/mL	Loading dose	0.5 mg	0.5 mg	50 mg	50 mg
	PCA dose	0.5 mg	0.5 mg	12 mg	25 mg
	Continuous	0.5 mg/hr	0.5 mg/hr	50 mg/hr	100 mg/hr
	Dose limit	None	None	100 mg	100 mg
	Time interval	1-hour period			
Fentanyl 50 mcg/mL	Loading dose	5 mcg	5 mcg	500 mcg	500 mcg
	PCA dose	5 mcg	5 mcg	125 mcg	250 mcg
	Continuous	5 mcg/hr	5 mcg/hr	500 mcg/hr	1000 mcg/hr
	Dose limit	None	None	1000 mcg	1000 mcg
	Time interval	1-hour period			

Source: Fairview Health Services, Hospira Lifecare PCA Pump Drug Library.

Table 6-4. Common PCA Dosing of Opioid Receptor Agonists

Drug	Demand Dose (PCA)	Continuous (Basal)	Lockout Interval
Morphine	1–2 mg	0–2 mg/hr	6–10 min
Hydromorphone	0.2–0.4 mg	0–0.4 mg/hr	6–10 min
Fentanyl	20–50 mcg	0–60 mcg/hr	5–10 min

Source: Grass JA. Patient controlled analgesia. *Anesth Analg.* 2005;101:S44-S61.

tive (refer to Table 6-3a). The total 1-hour dose limit should include the upper limits for both the loading and PCA doses.

The guidelines for IV PCA management are different for patients who are opioid tolerant and/or on chronic opioid therapy. Typically, the goal is to provide most (>80%) of the opioid requirements through a continuous infusion to meet the patient's chronic baseline and use larger PCA doses with longer lockout intervals for acute pain control.[2]

Continuous Infusion
Extreme caution is indicated in administering a continuous opioid infusion to opioid-naive patients, either as a sole infusion or in combination with PCA doses.[7] Most studies have failed to demonstrate any benefits when PCA is combined with a continuous infusion.[2]

Patients who are opioid-tolerant and/or are maintained on chronic opioids should receive a continuous infusion. In order to establish appropriate upper dose limits, a computer print-out of opioid infusions in different patients care areas (i.e., ICU, oncology, surgical units) is helpful in determining the maximum dose for each medication. High opioid doses may exceed the capacity of the PCA pump at standard concentrations (refer to Table 6-3b). A separate drug library for non-standard opioid concentrations may be needed for those patients.

Time Limits
The lockout interval is designed to prevent overdose. Ideally, it should be long enough for the patient to experience the maximal effect of one dose before another is permitted to prevent "dose stacking." Studies in literature indicate that the rate of distribution (flux) between the plasma and brain may be useful in determining the lockout interval.[2] Hence, the onset of peak analgesic effects may be useful in establishing the standard lockout interval.

A 10-minute lockout interval is commonly used for morphine and hydromorphone. Respiratory depression can occur in opioid naive patients with PCA doses of morphine >2 mg or hydromorphone >0.2 mg when the lockout interval is less than 10 minutes.[6] Standard order sets and institutional policies should limit the use of lockout intervals <10 minutes for morphine and hydromorphone unless recommended by a pain or anesthesia service. Patients with impaired renal or liver function may need a longer time interval between PCA doses in the range of 20–30 minutes for morphine and hydromorphone. Fentanyl requires a 5–8 minute lockout interval due to the need for frequent PCA dosing to accommodate for the rapid redistribution.[2]

Most PCA pumps have an option for a 1- or 4-hour time period for the upper limit for the total dose (refer to Table 6-3a and 6-3b).[7] The 1-hour period often requires more frequent monitoring of PCA use to adjust dosing as needed to control pain and side effects. For this reason, the 4-hour period is falling out of favor. Also, if the patient uses all the allotted doses early in the 4-hour period, this will lead to a long wait time before more pain medication can be administered via the PCA pump.[19]

Conclusion

There are several factors to consider when developing the PCA drug library. Patient safety recommendations, evidence-based guidelines, and institutional policies are major resources that should be used to establish upper and lower limits for each dose variable. The patient's level of opioid tolerance, clinical practice area, and nonstandard medications (i.e., investigational, non-opioid, etc.) may require the use of a separate drug library. A multidisciplinary process for development of the PCA drug library is fundamental to the understanding of the patient care, nursing, pharmacy and technology support requirements for this therapy.

PRACTICE TIPS

1. Review intravenous continuous infusion opioid doses in oncology patients. This may be useful in identifying the higher doses. Establishing upper hard limits for opioid tolerant patients should account for these high doses.
2. Review adverse event reports related to patient controlled analgesia doses in opioid naive patients. This information is useful for establishing upper hard limits based on safety data for this group of patients.
3. Limit the number of medications and concentrations based on frequency of use. Standard PCA medications and doses should be in a library that is easily recognizable by the nurse. Medications restricted to specialists (e.g., anesthesia) should be in a separate drug library.

References

1. Etches RC. Patient controlled analgesia. *Surg Clin North Am.* 1999;79(2):297-312.

2. Grass JA. Patient controlled analgesia. *Anesth Analg.* 2005;101:S44-S61.

3. Misprogramming PCA Concentration Leads to Dosing Errors. Institute for Safe Medication Practices Newsletter. August 28, 2008. Available at: http://www.ismp.org/newsletters.

4. Ladak SS, Chan VW, Easty T, Chagpar A. Right medication, right dose, right patient, right time, and right route: How do we select the right PCA device? *Pain Manag Nurs.* 2007;8(4):140-145.

5. Cohen MR, Smetzer J. Patient-controlled analgesia safety issues. *J Pain Palliat Care Pharmacother.* 2005;19(1)45-50.

6. Weber LM, Ghafoor VL, Phelps P. Implementation of standard order sets for patient-controlled analgesia. *Am J Health-Syst Pharm.* 2008;65:1184-1191.

7. Miaskowski C, Bair M, Chou R, D'Arcy Y, Hartwick C, et al. *Principles of Analgesic Use in the Treatment of Acute Pain and Cancer Pain.* 5th ed. Glenview, IL: American Pain Society; 2003.

8. Momeni M, Crucitti M, DeKock M. Patient-controlled analgesia in the management of postoperative pain. *Drugs.* 2006;18:2321-2337.

9. Stoelting RK. Opioid agonists and antagonists. In: Robert K. Stoelting, ed. *Pharmacology and Physiology in Anesthetic Practice.* 3rd ed. Philadelphia: Lippincott-Raven Publishers; 1999:77-112.

10. Sarhill N, Walsh D, Nelson KA. Hydromorphone: pharmacology and clinical applications in cancer patients. *Supportive Care Oncology.* 2001;9:84-96.

11. Murray A, Hagen N. Hydromorphone. *J Pain Symptom Manage.* 2005:29:S57-S66.

12. Peng PW, Sandler AN. A review of the use of fentanyl analgesia in the management of acute pain in adults. *Anesthesiology.* 1999;90:576-599.

13. Sweeney BP, Bromilow J. Liver enzyme induction and inhibition: implications for anaesthesia. *Anesthesia.* 2006;61:159-177.

14. Santiago-Palma J, Khojainova N, Kornick C, et al. Intravenous methadone in the management of chronic cancer pain. *Cancer.* 2001;92:1919-1925.

15. Shaiova L, Gerger A, Glinderman CD, et al. Consensus guideline on parenteral methadone use in pain and palliative care. *Palliative and Supportive Care.* 2008;6:165-176.

16. Krenn H, Oxzanski W, Jellinek H, et al. Nalbuphine by PCA-pump for analgesia following hysterectomy: bolus application versus continuous infusion with bolus application. *European J Pain.* 2001;5:219-226.

17. Proceedings of a summit on preventing patient harm and death from IV medication errors. *Am J Health-Syst Pharm.* 2008;65:2367-2379.

18. Ginsberg B, Latta KS. Acute pain management. Arthur G. Lipman, ed. *Pain Management for Primary Care Clinicians.* Bethesda, MD: American Society of Health-System Pharmacists; 2004.

19. D'Arcy Y. Keep your patient safe during PCA. *Nursing.* 2008;50-55. Available at: www.nursing2008.com.

Building a Pediatric Drug Library

Melissa K. Carlson and Angela Skoglund

Key Terms

Adult patient—a patient 17 years old and weighing at least 45 kilograms.

Drug library subset—a subset of the larger drug library that includes all drugs needed for a specific patient population or area. Other names that pump vendors use for these subsets are personalities, profiles, and clinical care areas.

Large volume pump—an infusion device used to deliver medications for which a very small volume or rate of infusion is not necessary.

Neonatal patient—a patient less than 1 month old.

Pediatric patient—a patient older than 1 month but younger than 17 years and weighing less than 45 kilograms.

Smart infusion pumps—a new generation of infusion pumps that incorporates dose limiting software into the pump hardware; this software is designed to prevent infusion-related programming errors. The Joint Commission, in the 2006 National Patient Safety Goals, defined a smart pump as a "parenteral infusion pump equipped with IV medication error-prevention software that alerts operators or interrupts the infusion process when a pump setting is programmed outside of pre-configured limits." Smart pumps are designed to recognize prescription errors, dose misinterpretations, and keypad programming errors.

Syringe pump—an infusion device used to deliver medications that require a very small volume or rate of infusion.

Introduction

Medication errors are more likely to occur with pediatric patients than with adult patients, due to the necessity of using individualized dosage calculations in this population.[1-3] Specifically at risk are children in pediatric intensive care units, neonatal intensive care units, oncology units, and in the emergency department.[3] The use of intelligent infusion devices along with standard medication concentrations has been shown to reduce errors associated with continuous infusions in pediatric patients by up to 73%.[1]

Intelligent infusion device technology allows for programming of customized drug libraries that can be geared specifically for this high-risk group of patients. Unlike medications for adult patients, medications for pediatric patients are often dosed based on the patient-specific weight. Use of these intelligent infusion devices can eliminate the need for weight-based calculations, force the use of standard concentrations and dosing units, alert practitioners to potential programming or dosing errors, and track instances where alerts are overridden or bypassed, thereby defeating the built-in safety features of the device. This chapter will discuss the many factors which must be considered in order to design appropriate drug libraries for pediatric patients.

Defining Drug Library Subsets for Pediatrics

Most pediatric hospitals care for a wide range of pediatric patients. Patients housed on pediatric units requiring the use of an infusion device could range in weight from less than 500 grams to greater than 100 kilograms. Furthermore, pediatric services may encompass many types of patient care areas, such as neonatal intensive care (NICU), pediatric intensive care (PICU), pediatric hematology/oncology, pediatric surgery, pediatric general medicine, pediatric bone marrow transplant, newborn nursery, pediatric sedation, and pediatric emergency services.

Intravenous infusion practices may be highly variable between pediatric patient populations or patient care areas, even within the same hospital or care system. Often, misperceptions exist that a certain area is unique and will not be able to standardize practice in such a way as to make intelligent infusion device use possible. It is essential that hospitals evaluate how infusion devices are currently being used in these settings in order to help define appropriate drug library subsets that meet the needs of each patient population or patient care unit.[4] Interdisciplinary participation in this evaluation is crucial in order to effectively assess all aspects of the infusion practice spectrum and develop support for these safety enhancements.

In pediatric practice, it is common for some medications to be infused via a syringe pump while others may be infused via a large volume pump. Often, the choice of infusion device will directly relate to the actual medication dose prescribed and/or the age and weight of the patient. In many cases, guidelines may need to be established by the hospital as to when a certain type of infusion device will be used. These guidelines may address patient weight, patient age, or patient location. There will need to be a firm definition for what weight and age constitutes a pediatric patient versus an adult patient and how the library subsets are utilized. Our institution uses a weight cutoff of 45 kilograms to differentiate between adult and pediatric patients for the purpose of drug libraries. Furthermore, guidelines may regulate the use of an infusion device with regard to a specific medication or address limitations regarding the lowest dose the infusion device is able to deliver, based on the institution's standard concentration of a medication. One example of this in our institution is a policy where insulin is only delivered on a syringe pump, regardless of patient age or unit.

Neonatal patients, defined as less than 1 month of age, generally receive most infusions via a syringe pump because these patients require very small medication doses which can often not be delivered by a large volume pump. A large volume pump drug library for a NICU patient population would likely require a much smaller list of medications and IV fluids to be present than that for a PICU population, which would include larger patients. Since these two patient care areas have differing needs, it may make sense to assign separate drug library subsets within the large volume infusion device for each area. This prevents the practitioners in the NICU from having extraneous medication options to scroll through, thereby reducing the chance of a drug selection error.

Drug library subsets may also be broken down by weight. For example, libraries could be built for "Peds 0–5 kg," "Peds 6–10 kg," "Peds 11–20 kg," "Peds 21–30 kg," "Peds 31–40 kg," and "Peds 41–50 kg." This type of drug library subset arrangement may allow for the programming of much more restrictive dosing limits, which may improve safety for high-risk, low therapeutic index medications. The down side to developing multiple weight-based drug library subsets is that this configuration adds more complexity to the overall library.

Different types and models of infusion devices offer diverse options with regard to available delivery modes, infusion units, and dose limits. Some devices allow the selection of specific parameters for different library subsets. One example of this is alarm volume. Our institution was able to select a lower alarm volume for our NICU libraries than for the other pediatric libaries. Other options may include setting a specific maximum infusion rate (without respect to dose) for an entire library subset or the ability to program a maximum total dose for a given medication within a subset. Thoughtful utilization of these types of options can add another level of safety to the library system.

Institutions using multiple types of infusion devices will need to decide whether differences in drug libraries are required between devices. For instance, our institution uses a combination of syringe pumps and large volume infusion devices for pediatric patients. As a result of differing technological capabilities, the corresponding medication libraries are somewhat different. Therefore, examples of both large volume infusion device libraries and syringe pump libraries will be provided.

Some infusion devices allow for the configuration of sub-library categories within a specific library subset. At our institution, we chose to use this feature with our syringe pumps to create alphabetical groupings of medications within each library, thus decreasing the amount of scrolling required by the nurse when programming the device. We also considered grouping chemotherapy given via the syringe pump within a separate sub-library group.

The actual number of pediatric drug library subsets developed by an institution will depend largely on how variable current infusion practices are, the types of pediatric patients cared for by the institution, and the capabilities of the infusion device that the institution has chosen to purchase. There is no right or wrong number, but the risks and benefits with different approaches need to be weighed. As more pediatric drug library subsets are created, the potential for the practitioner to make an incorrect choice during programming increases. In order to prevent this from happening, close attention should be paid to the naming of pediatric drug library subsets to make it easy for practitioners to select the appropriate subset for their patient. It is advisable to adopt a specific naming convention that is standard across each library subset. Infusion devices do generally have a character limit for subset names, which can make this task difficult (see Tables 7-1, 7-2, and 7-3).

Defining a Medication List for Each Pediatric Drug Library Subset

Once the pediatric drug library subsets have been defined, a list of medications to be included in each library will need to be developed. Data should be obtained regarding the most common infusions used in each area to help guide medication selection. This may include both continuous infusions and intermittent infusions. Furthermore, if the selected infusion device does not allow for medications to be given outside of a library, a focus group should be convened to brainstorm all

Table 7-1. Pediatric Large Volume Infusion Device Drug Library Subset Examples

Library Example #1	Library Example #2	Library Example #3
PedsGen	0–5 kg	NICU 0–5 kg
PICU	6–10 kg	PICU 6–20 kg
NICU	11–20 kg	PICU 21–45 kg
PedsBMT	21–30 kg	PedsGen 6–20 kg
ChemoBio	21–30 kg	PedsGen 21–45 kg
	41–50 kg	PedsBMT
	ChemoBio	ChemoBio

Table 7-2. Syringe Pump Drug Library Subset Example
Library Example
NICU – Continuous
NICU – Intermittent
PICU – Continuous
PICU – Intermittent
PedsGen – Continuous
PedsGen – Intermittent
Peds Chemotherapy
Anesthesia
Adult ICU
Adult MedSurg
OB

Table 7-3. Syringe Pump Sub-Library Example
PICU – Intermittent Library
PICU A
PICU B–Ce
PICU Ch–E
PICU F–G
PICU H–L
PICU M–Pe
PICU Ph–Q
PICU R–Z

possible medications that may need to be given via each library subset in order to make sure that patient care will not be compromised by implementation of the new device. A generic drug entry, such as "Other Drug" should also be considered. Naming of the medications within the pump should be done in a standardized method. Use of tallman lettering is recommended to improve safety by reducing selection errors. In the future, bar-coding technology should further reduce the risk of these types of errors. The order in which the medication names appear in the pump library is also up to the design committee. Medications can be listed alphabetically, by frequency of use, or some combination thereof. In the large volume device examples provided, several commonly used medications are listed first, followed by an alphabetical listing. This prevents the nurse from having to scroll through many medications for common items, such as generic IV fluids. It should be noted that the large volume device examples included below do not contain opioid or insulin drips, as our institution currently infuses these agents on different infusion devices (see Tables 7-4, 7-5, 7-6, and 7-7).

Establishing Standard Concentrations

Whenever possible, standard concentrations should be designated for continuous infusions. Concentrations should be chosen based on published administration guidelines, volume considerations, stability information, and compatibility information. Standard concentrations delivered via intelligent infusion device technology not only eliminate the need for individualized dosage and rate calculations, but also simplify the preparation of the product for the pharmacy. Another benefit to standard concentrations is simplified ordering of infusions by the prescriber. In most cases, intelligent infusion devices will allow the programmer to make continuous infusion dose adjustments directly, without performing any calculations.[1]

Table 7-4. Large Volume Infusion Device Library Subset Medication List Example #1

PICU

- Aminocaproic acid drip
- Bumetanide drip
- Dexmedetomidine drip
- Dopamine drip
- Epinephrine drip
- Heparin drip
- Midazolam drip
- Milrinone drip
- Nitroprusside (+ sodium thiosulfate) drip
- Norepinephrine drip
- Propofol drip
- Vecuronium drip
- IV fluid
- IV fluid + KCl
- TPN
- Lipid 20%
- 3% sodium chloride
- 23.4% sodium chloride
- Acetylcysteine dose
- Alprostadil drip
- Alteplase drip
- Aminophylline drip
- Amiodarone drip
- Antibiotic 50 mL
- Antibiotic 100 mL
- Antibiotic 150 mL
- Antibiotic 250 mL
- Antibiotic 500 mL
- Calcium chloride replacement dose
- PRISMA calcium chloride drip
- Calcium gluconate replacement dose
- Calcium gluconate drip
- Cisatracurium drip
- Cycle fluid
- Cyclosporine drip
- Cyclosporine intermittent dose
- Dantrolene drip
- Diltiazem drip
- Dobutamine drip
- Esmolol drip
- Fosphenytoin dose
- Furosemide drip
- Immune globulin dose
- Isoproterenol drip
- K cocktail adult
- K cocktail pediatric
- Ketamine drip
- Labetalol drip
- Lepirudin drip
- Lidocaine drip
- Lorazepam drip
- Magnesium sulfate replacement dose
- Methylprednisolone drip
- Mycophenolate intermittent dose
- Naloxone drip
- Nesiritide drip
- Nitroglycerin drip
- Octreotide drip
- Ondansetron drip
- Other drug
- Pantoprazole drip
- Pentobarbital drip
- Phenylephrine drip
- Piperacillin/tazobactam continuous infusion
- Potassium chloride replacement dose
- Procainamide drip
- Potassium phosphate replacement dose
- Sodium bicarbonate drip
- Sodium phosphate replacement dose
- Tacrolimus drip
- Theophylline drip
- Thymoglobulin dose
- Vancomycin dose
- Vasopressin drip

One disadvantage of standard concentrations in the pediatric population is that they may limit the prescriber's choice of fluid volume that is delivered to the patient. This may especially be of concern in an NICU population, where patients are very small and fluid management is very precise. This limitation can be overcome with careful selection of standard concentrations. For some medications, it may be warranted to select multiple standard concentrations, although the Institute for Safe Medication Practices recommends a limit of two concentrations per medication[5] (see Tables 7-8 and 7-9).

Table 7-5. Large Volume Infusion Device Library Subset Medication List Example #2

PedsGen

- IV fluid
- IV fluid + KCl
- TPN
- Cycle fluid
- Lipid 20%
- Heparin drip
- 3% sodium chloride
- Acetylcysteine dose
- Aminophylline drip
- Antibiotic 50 mL
- Antibiotic 100 mL
- Antibiotic 150 mL
- Antibiotic 250 mL
- Antibiotic 500 mL
- Calcium gluconate replacement dose
- Cyclosporine drip
- Cyclosporine intermittent dose
- Fosphenytoin dose
- Immune globulin dose
- K cocktail adult
- K cocktail pediatric
- Ketamine drip
- Lepirudin drip
- Magnesium sulfate replacement dose
- Mycophenolate intermittent dose
- Naloxone drip
- Octreotide drip
- Ondansetron drip
- Other drug
- Pantoprazole drip
- Piperacillin/tazobactam continuous infusion
- Potassium chloride replacement dose
- Potassium phosphate replacement dose
- Sodium bicarbonate drip
- Sodium phosphate replacement dose
- Tacrolimus drip
- Theophylline drip
- Thymoglobulin dose
- Vancomycin dose

Table 7-6. Large Volume Infusion Device Library Subset Medication List Example #3

NICU

- TPN
- IV fluid
- IV fluid + KCl
- Cycle fluid
- Heparin drip
- Heparin drip
- K cocktail neonatal
- Other drug

Establishing Dosing Units and Limits

Following identification of the appropriate medications for each library subset, decisions will need to be made regarding standard dosing units and dosing limits will need to be defined for each medication. The dosing limits should be tailored specifically to the patient population that will be using each library subset and to the prescribing habits of physicians at your institution.

Standard dosing units should be chosen based on best practices in pediatrics. Using the dosing units that the medication is commonly ordered in eliminates the need for the programmer to perform any calculations when setting up the pump. However, there are often multiple options for how a medication could be delivered on an infusion device. One example of this is vecuronium, where the dosing units could be programmed in either mg/kg/hr or mcg/kg/min. When thinking about which dosing units to choose, be sure to consider both current practice and patient safety. In large teaching hospitals that serve both pediatric patients and adult patients, there are often medical residents rotating through both adult and pediatric areas. If the standard dosing units programmed for a particular

Table 7-7. Syringe Pump Library Subset Medication List Examples

NICU—Continuous	PICU—Continuous	PICU—Intermittent	GenPeds—Continuous	GenPeds—Intermittent	Anesthesia	Adult ICU	Adult MedSurg	OB
Alprostadil	Alprostadil	Abelcet	Aminophylline	Abelcet	Propofol	Epoprostenol	Epoprostenol	Insulin, regular
Aminocaproic acid	Alteplase	Acetylcysteine	Argatroban	Acetylcysteine	Remifentanil	Insulin, regular	Insulin, regular	
Aminophylline	Aminocaproic acid	Acetazolamide	Bumetanide	Acetazolamide	Sufentanil	Propofol	Treprostinil	
Bumetanide	Aminophylline	Acyclovir	Calcium gluconate	Acyclovir		Treprostinil		
Calcium gluconate	Ammonal	Albumin	Deferoxamine	Albumin				
Cisatracurium	Argatroban	Amikacin	Epoprostenol	Amikacin				
Dexmedetomidine	Arginine	Aminophylline	Fentanyl	Aminophylline				
Dobutamine	Bumetanide	Amphotericin B	Furosemide	Amphotericin B				
Dopamine	Calcium chloride	Ampicillin	Heparin	Ampicillin				
Epinephrine	Calcium gluconate	Ampicillin/ sulbactam	Hydromorphone	Ampicillin/ sulbactam				
Epoprostenol	Cisatracurium	Anti-thrombin III	Insulin, regular	Azathioprine				
Esmolol	Deferoxamine	Azathioprine	Intralipid	Azithromycin				
Fentanyl	Dexmedetomidine	Azithromycin	IV Solution	Aztreonam				
Heparin	Diltiazem	Aztreonam	Lepirudin	Bumetanide				
Hydromorphone	Dobutamine	Bumetanide	Morphine	Caffeine citrate				
Insulin, regular	Dopamine	Caffeine citrate	Octreotide	Calcium gluconate				
Intralipid	Epinephrine	Calcium chloride	Ondansetron	Carnitine				
Isoproterenol	Epoprostenol	Calcium gluconate	Pantoprazole	Caspofungin				
IV Solution	Esmolol	Carnitine	Sodium bicarbonate	Cefazolin				
Labetalol	Fentanyl	Caspofungin	Theophylline	Cefepime				
Lidocaine	Furosemide	Cefazolin	Treprostinil	Cefotaxime				
Midazolam	Heparin	Cefepime		Cefoxitin				
Milrinone	Hydromorphone	Cefotaxime		Ceftazidime				
Morphine	Insulin, regular	Cefoxitin		Ceftriaxone				
Nitroglycerin	Intralipid	Ceftazidime		Cefuroxime				
Nitroprusside	Isoproterenol	Ceftriaxone		Chloramphenicol				
Norepinephrine	IV Solution	Cefuroxime		Chlorothiazide				
Octreotide	Ketamine	Chloramphenicol						
	Labetalol							

Continued

Table 7-7. Syringe Pump Library Subset Medication List Examples [cont'd]

NICU—Continuous	PICU—Continuous	PICU—Intermittent	GenPeds—Continuous	GenPeds—Intermittent	Anesthesia	Adult ICU	Adult MedSurg	OB
Ondansetron	Lepirudin	Chlorothiazide		Ciprofloxacin				
Pantoprazole	Lidocaine	Ciprofloxacin		Clindamycin				
Phenylephrine	Lorazepam	Clindamycin		Desmopressin				
Potassium	Methylprednisolone	Desmopressin		Dexamethasone				
Procainamide	Midazolam	Dexamethasone		Digoxin				
Propofol	Milrinone	Digoxin		Diltiazem				
Sodium bicarbonate	Morphine	Diltiazem		Diphenhydramine				
Vasopressin	Nesiritide	Diphenhydramine		Doxycycline				
Vecuronium	Nicardipine	Doxycycline		Enalaprilat				
	Nitroglycerin	Enalaprilat		Epoetin alfa				
	Nitroprusside	Epoetin alfa		Erythromycin lactobionate				
	Norepinephrine	Erythromycin lactobionate		Fentanyl				
	Octreotide	Fentanyl		Filgrastim				
	Ondansetron	Filgrastim		Fluconazole				
	Pantoprazole	Fluconazole		Foscarnet				
	Pentobarbital	Foscarnet		Fosphenytoin				
	Phenylephrine	Fosphenytoin		Furosemide				
	Procainamide	Furosemide		Ganciclovir				
	Propofol	Ganciclovir		Gentamicin				
	Sodium bicarbonate	Gentamicin		Glycopyrrolate				
	Theophylline	Glycopyrrolate		Granisetron				
	Treprostinil	Granisetron		Hydralazine				
	Vasopressin	Hydralazine		Hydrocortisone				
	Vecuronium	Hydrocortisone		Hydromorphone				
		Hydromorphone		Hydroxyzine				
		Hydroxyzine		Imipenem/cilastatin				
		Imipenem/cilastatin		Ketorolac				

Continued

Table 7-7. Syringe Pump Library Subset Medication List Examples [cont'd]

NICU—Continuous	PICU—Continuous	PICU—Intermittent	GenPeds—Continuous	GenPeds—Intermittent	Anesthesia	Adult ICU	Adult MedSurg	OB
		Ketorolac		Labetalol				
		Labetalol		Levofloxacin				
		Levofloxacin		Levothyroxine				
		Levothyroxine		Linezolid				
		Linezolid		Lorazepam				
		Lorazepam		Magnesium sulfate				
		Magnesium sulfate		Meropenem				
		Meropenem		Methadone				
		Methadone		Methylprednisolone				
		Methylprednisolone		Metoclopramide				
		Metoclopramide		Metronidazole				
		Metronidazole		Midazolam				
		Midazolam		Morphine				
		Morphine		Mycophenolate				
		Mycophenolate		Nafcillin				
		Nafcillin		Octreotide				
		Octreotide		Ondansetron				
		Ondansetron		Pantoprazole				
		Pantoprazole		Penicillin GK				
		Penicillin GK		Pentamidine				
		Pentamidine		Phytonadione				
		Phenobarbital		Piperacillin				
		Phytonadione		Piperacillin/tazobactam				
		Piperacillin		Potassium chloride				
		Piperacillin/tazobactam		Prochlorperazine				
		Potassium chloride		Promethazine				
		Prochlorperazine		Propranolol				

Continued

Table 7-7. Syringe Pump Library Subset Medication List Examples (cont'd)

NICU—Continuous	PICU—Continuous	PICU—Intermittent	GenPeds—Continuous	GenPeds—Intermittent	Anesthesia	Adult ICU	Adult MedSurg	OB
		Promethazine		Quinupristin/				
		Propranolol		Dalfopristin				
		Quinupristin/		Ranitidine				
		Dalfopristin		Rifampin				
		Ranitidine		Sodium				
		Rifampin		bicarbonate				
		Sodium		Ticarcillin/				
		Bicarbonate		clavulanate				
		Ticarcillin/		Tobramycin				
		Clavulanate		TMP/				
		Tobramycin		sulfamethoxazole				
		TMP/		Valproate				
		Sulfamethoxazole		Vancomycin				
		Tromethamine		Voriconazole				
		Valproate						
		Vancomycin						
		Voriconazole						

medication infusion are different between these populations, it may lead to a programming error if the medication order was written in the wrong dosing units for that area. In our institution, we found that the prevailing practice in pediatrics was to order vecuronium and cisatracurium as mg/kg/hr while the adult services ordered them in mcg/kg/min. After much discussion, we chose to standardize across the entire hospital to mcg/kg/min. We provided physicians and nurses with the following reference cards until they became accustomed to the new dosing units.

Using weight-based dosing units in pediatrics (i.e., mg/kg/hr, mcg/kg/min, etc.) when possible is generally accepted as a safer way to deliver medications. Medications programmed in mL/hr, mg/dose, or mg/day will require a much larger window of acceptable dose values if the patient population for a particular library subset ranges greatly in weight.

Education may need to be completed for nurses and physicians around standard dosing units.

Table 7-8. Standard Concentrations for Continuous Infusions[6–12]

Medication	Standard Concentration	Other Concentrations Available in Pump
Alprostadil	0.01 mg/mL (10 mcg/mL)	
Aminophylline	2 mg/mL	
Aminocaproic acid	50 mg/mL	
Amiodarone	1 mg/mL	6 mg/mL
Bumetanide	0.25 mg/mL (250 mcg/mL)	0.125 mg/mL (125 mcg/mL)
Calcium chloride	100 mg/mL	8 mg/mL (PRISMA)
Calcium gluconate	50 mg/mL	
Cisatracurium	2 mg/mL	
Cyclosporine	1 mg/mL	
Dantrolene	0.33 mg/mL	
Dexmedetomidine	0.004 mg/mL (4 mcg/mL)	
Diltiazem	1 mg/mL	
Dobutamine	2 mg/mL	5 mg/mL
Dopamine	1.6 mg/mL	3.2 mg/mL, 6.4 mg/mL
Epinephrine	0.02 mg/mL (20 mcg/mL)	0.04 mg/mL (40 mcg/mL), 0.064 mg/mL (64 mcg/mL)
Esmolol	20 mg/mL	10 mg/mL
Furosemide	1 mg/mL	
Heparin	100 units/mL	
Isoproterenol	0.02 mg/mL (20 mcg/mL)	
Ketamine	2 mg/mL	
Labetalol	5 mg/mL	
Lepirudin	0.4 mg/mL	
Lidocaine	8 mg/mL	
Lorazepam	1 mg/mL	
Midazolam	1 mg/mL	0.5 mg/mL
Milrinone	0.2 mg/mL	
Naloxone	0.04 mg/mL (40 mcg/mL)	
Nesiritide	0.006 mg/mL (6 mcg/mL)	
Nicardipine	0.1 mg/mL	0.4 mg/mL
Nitroglycerin	0.2 mg/mL	
Nitroprusside (+ sodium thiosulfate)	0.4 mg/mL (+ 4 mg/mL)	1.6 mg/mL (+ 16 mg/mL)
Norepinephrine	0.032 mg/mL (32 mcg/mL)	0.064 mg/mL (64 mcg/mL)
Octreotide	0.005 mg/mL (5 mcg/mL)	
Ondansetron	1 mg/mL	
Pantoprazole	0.8 mg/mL	
Pentobarbital	8 mg/mL	
Phenylephrine	0.2 mg/mL	
Procainamide	8 mg/mL	

Continued

Table 7-8. Standard Concentrations for Continuous Infusions[6-12] [cont'd]

Medication	Standard Concentration	Other Concentrations Available in Pump
Propofol	10 mg/mL	
Ranitidine	1 mg/mL	
Sodium bicarbonate	1 mEq/mL	
Tacrolimus	0.02 mg/mL (20 mcg/mL)	
Theophylline	1.6 mg/mL	
Vasopressin	1 unit/mL	
Vecuronium	1 mg/mL	

When bumetanide was added to intelligent infusion devices at our institution, physicians were expected to order the drug as mcg/kg/hr versus the conventional mg/kg/day. Again, we provided physicians and nurses with reference cards until they became accustomed to the new dosing units.

Dosing alerts should be based on usual and maximum doses published in pediatric reference books and the primary literature. Soft limits may be set to alert the staff member programming the pump that the dose exceeds the usual dose for that patient population. These alerts allow the staff member to override, if indicated. Hard limits are more often programmed to alert the staff to "catastrophic" doses, many that may result from an extra keystroke or misplaced decimal. These alerts force reprogramming of the pump. It is not usually required to program a low hard, low soft, high hard, and high soft limit for each drug. Pros and cons as to which types of limits are ultimately set should be considered on a drug by drug basis. For instance, if a low hard limit is not set for a particular drug, by default, the lowest dose that can be delivered will be based on the lowest infusion rate that the pump capable of. In our case, this is 0.1 mL/hr for our large volume device. As shown in Tables 7-7 through 7-10, our institution utilized both soft and hard limits. We agreed upon a standard method for calculating these limits. Our soft limits were determined by multiplying the low and high usual doses by 0.9 (low soft) and the 1.1 (high soft). This method should allow for prescriber rounding of doses. The hard limits were determined by multiplying the low and high usual doses by 0.1 (low hard) and 1.2 (high hard). We felt that these limits would prevent accidental decimal calculation errors that might lead to a catastrophic under or overdose (see Table 7-11).

Many pumps also feature a bolus dose option. Use of this option is important to consider in pediatrics. Depending on the infusion device, limits can be placed on medication boluses by dose, dose per kilogram, rate of administration, and/or time for administration. Tables 7-12 and 7-13 provide examples of possible dosing limit schemes. Some infusion software may allow the nurse to input a dose as a straight number of milligrams and is still able to accept limits programmed in milligrams per kilogram. This was not possible with the device selected at our

Table 7-9. Standard Concentrations for Pediatric Intermittent Infusions[6–12]

Medication	Standard Concentration	Other Concentrations Available in Pump
Abelcet	2 mg/mL	
Acetazolamide	100 mg/mL	20 mg/mL
Acetylcysteine	40 mg/mL	
Acyclovir	5 mg/mL	
Albumin	5 mg/mL (5%)	25 mg/mL (25%)
Amikacin	5 mg/mL	
Aminophylline	25 mg/mL	100 mg/mL
Amphotericin B	0.1 mg/mL	0.25 mg/mL
Ampicillin	25 mg/mL	250 mg/mL
Ampicillin/sulbactam	45 mg/mL	
Azathioprine	10 mg/mL	
Azithromycin	2 mg/mL	
Aztreonam	20 mg/mL	
Bumetanide	0.25 mg/mL	0.125 mg/mL
Caffeine citrate	10 mg/mL	
Calcium chloride	100 mg/mL	20 mg/mL
Calcium gluconate	50 mg/mL	100 mg/mL
Carnitine	100 mg/mL	
Caspofungin	0.5 mg/mL	
Cefazolin	50 mg/mL	100 mg/mL
Cefepime	40 mg/mL	
Cefotaxime	40 mg/mL	150 mg/mL
Cefoxitin	40 mg/mL	
Ceftazidime	40 mg/mL	200 mg/mL
Ceftriaxone	40 mg/mL	
Cefuroxime	50 mg/mL	
Chloramphenicol	20 mg/mL	
Chlorothiazide	25 mg/mL	
Ciprofloxacin	2 mg/mL	
Clindamycin	18 mg/mL	
Desmopressin	0.5 mcg/mL	
Dexamethasone	4 mg/mL	1 mg/mL
Digoxin	50 mcg/mL	5 mcg/mL
Diltiazem	5 mg/mL	
Diphenhydramine	50 mg/mL	2 mg/mL
Doxycycline	1 mg/mL	
Enalaprilat	1,250 mcg/mL	25 mcg/mL
Epoetin alfa	10,000 units/mL	
Erythromycin lactobionate	5 mg/mL	

Continued

Table 7-9. Standard Concentrations for Pediatric Intermittent Infusions[6–12] (cont'd)

Medication	Standard Concentration	Other Concentrations Available in Pump
Fentanyl	50 mcg/mL	
Filgrastim	15 mcg/mL	
Fluconazole	2 mg/mL	
Foscarnet	12 mg/mL	24 mg/mL
Fosphenytoin	5 mg/mL	25 mg/mL
Furosemide	10 mg/mL	2 mg/mL
Ganciclovir	5 mg/mL	
Gentamicin	10 mg/mL	
Glycopyrrolate	200 mcg/mL	25 mcg/mL
Granisetron	1 mg/mL	
Hydralazine	20 mg/mL	2 mg/mL
Hydrocortisone	50 mg/mL	2 mg/mL
Hydromorphone	1 mg/mL	
Hydroxyzine	1 mg/mL	25 mg/mL
Imipenem/cilastatin	5 mg/mL	
Indomethacin	0.5 mg/mL	
Ketorolac	15 mg/mL	
Labetalol	5 mg/mL	2 mg/mL
Leucovorin	10 mg/mL	
Levofloxacin	5 mg/mL	
Levothyroxine	40 mcg/mL	
Linezolid	2 mg/mL	
Magnesium sulfate	100 mg/mL	25 mg/mL
Meropenem	50 mg/mL	
Mesna	100 mg/mL	
Methadone	1 mg/mL	10 mg/mL
Methylprednisolone	40 mg/mL	2 mg/mL
Metoclopramide	0.5 mg/mL	
Metronidazole	5 mg/mL	
Midazolam	1 mg/mL	
Mycophenolate	6 mg/mL	
Nafcillin	40 mg/mL	
Octreotide	100 mcg/mL	
Ondansetron	2 mg/mL	
Pantoprazole	4 mg/mL	
Penicillin GK	100,000 units/mL	
Pentamidine	2 mg/mL	
Phenobarbital	10 mg/mL	65 mg/mL
Phytonadione	0.2 mg/mL	

Continued

Table 7-9. Standard Concentrations for Pediatric Intermittent Infusions[6–12] (cont'd)

Medication	Standard Concentration	Other Concentrations Available in Pump
Piperacillin	20 mg/mL	
Piperacillin/tazobactam	45 mg/mL	
Potassium chloride	0.1 mEq/mL	0.4 mEq/mL, 1 mEq/mL (PICU/NICU)
Prochlorperazine	5 mg/mL	
Promethazine	2.5 mg/mL	
Propranolol	1 mg/mL	0.01 mg/mL
Quinupristin/dalfopristin	2 mg/mL	5 mg/mL
Ranitidine	2.5 mg/mL	
Rifampin	6 mg/mL	
Sodium bicarbonate	0.5 mEq/mL	1 mEq/mL
Ticarcillin/clavulanate	31 mg/mL	
Tobramycin	10 mg/mL	
Tromethamine	0.3 mMol/mL	
Valproate	10 mg/mL	
Vancomycin	2.5 mg/mL	5 mg/mL, 10 mg/mL
Voriconazole	5 mg/mL	
Zidovudine	4 mg/mL	

Vecuronium Dose Conversion Chart

Dose in mg/kg/hr	Equivalent Dose in mcg/kg/min
0.06 mg/kg/hr	1 mcg/kg/min
0.09 mg/kg/hr	1.5 mcg/kg/min
0.12 mg/kg/hr	2 mcg/kg/min
0.15 mg/kg/hr	2.5 mcg/kg/min

Figure 7-1. Vecuronium reference card.

Cisatracurium Dose Conversion Chart

Dose in mg/kg/hr	Equivalent Dose in mcg/kg/min
0.06 mg/kg/hr	1 mcg/kg/min
0.09 mg/kg/hr	1.5 mcg/kg/min
0.12 mg/kg/hr	2 mcg/kg/min
0.15 mg/kg/hr	2.5 mcg/kg/min
0.18 mg/kg/hr	3 mcg/kg/min
0.21 mg/kg/hr	3.5 mcg/kg/min

Figure 7-2. Cisatracurium reference card.

Bumetanide Dose Conversion Chart

Daily Dose	Equivalent Dose in mcg/kg/hr
0.35 mg/kg/day	14.6 mcg/kg/hr
0.3 mg/kg/day	12.5 mcg/kg/hr
0.25 mg/kg/day	10.4 mcg/kg/hr
0.2 mg/kg/day	8.3 mcg/kg/hr

Figure 7-3. Bumetanide reference card.

institution. At our site, bolus doses are generally not ordered as a weight-based dose. Instead, one is more likely to see a physician write an order such as "Give an additional 250 units of heparin now" or "Give 250 units of heparin now, and then start an infusion at 20 units/kg/hr." In our case, if you program the bolus dose limits on a device in a weight-based fashion (i.e., low hard limit of 10 units/ kg and high hard limit of 60 units/kg), these will be the units that the device will expect the nurse to use to enter the dose during programming. In this example, because the original order was not written as a weight-based dose, the nurse would have to perform a calculation in order to program the pump. When non-weight-based limits are programmed in to the bolus feature, the range of acceptable doses becomes very wide for patient populations with varying weights. A PICU library intended for patients 6–45 kilograms that uses non-weight based bolus limits would require an acceptable dose range of something like 60–2700 units for a medication like heparin. In this instance, library subsets with tighter weight ranges would likely be safer. Another option is to consider changing practice around how these medications are ordered by requiring weight-based bolus dose orders.

Conclusion

Intelligent infusion devices can reduce the frequency of medication errors in a pediatric setting. They allow for customization of drug libraries and dosing alerts for this high-risk population. Due consideration should be given to each of the many factors that must be considered for pediatric library development, as implementation of this technology in a thoughtful manner can avert potentially life-threatening events.

<u>Disclaimer:</u> Dosing limits should be based upon hospital utilization patterns, as well as acceptable dosing ranges. Some of the dosing limits presented here exceed FDA-approved doses. This was done to avoid excessive alerts and alert fatigue. Use caution when deciding appropriate dosing limits.

Table 7-10. PICU Large Volume Infusion Device and Syringe Pump Continuous Infusion Dosing Limits[6, 13–17]

Medication	Infusion Mode	Low Hard Limit	Low Soft Limit	High Soft Limit	High Hard Limit
23.4% sodium chloride[a]	mL/hr	None	None	None	180
3% sodium chloride	mL/hr	None	None	None	90
Acetylcysteine – renal Protocol	mL/hr	None	None	400	None
Acetylcysteine step 1 ___g / 200 mL	mL/hr	None	None	None	200
Acetylcysteine step 2 ___g / 500 mL	mL/hr	None	None	None	125
Acetylcysteine step 3 ___g / 1000 mL	mL/hr	None	None	None	62.5
Albumin 25%	mL/hr	None	0.1	60	None
Albumin 5%	mL/hr	None	0.1	240	None
Alprostadil drip 0.01 mg/mL	mcg/kg/min	None	0.05	0.1	0.4
Aminocaproic acid drip 50 mg/mL	mg/kg/hr	None	None	33.3	34
Aminophylline drip 2 mg/mL	mg/kg/hr	None	0.5	1.2	1.5
Amiodarone drip (max) 6 mg/mL	mcg/kg/min	None	5	None	15
Amiodarone drip (std) 1 mg/mL	mcg/kg/min	None	5	None	15
Antibiotic 100 mL	mL/hr	None	50	400	None
Antibiotic 150 mL	mL/hr	None	75	150	None
Antibiotic 250 mL	mL/hr	None	125	250	None
Antibiotic 50 mL	mL/hr	None	25	200	None
Antibiotic 500 mL	mL/hr	None	100	500	None
Bumetanide drip (low) 0.125 mg/mL[b]	mcg/kg/hr	None	4	15	16.5
Bumetanide drip (std) 0.25 mg/mL[b]	mcg/kg/hr	None	4	15	16.5
Calcium chloride drip 100 mg/mL	mg/hr	None	None	375	400
Calcium chloride drip PRISMA 8 mg/mL	mL/hr	None	None	30	None
Calcium chloride replacement 100 mg/mL	mL/hr	None	0.1	40	None
Calcium gluconate drip 100 mg/mL	mg/hr	None	None	950	1000
Calcium gluconate replacement 50 mg/mL	mL/hr	None	0.1	120	None
Cisatracurium drip 2 mg/mL	mcg/kg/min	None	1	3	4
Cycle fluid	mL/hr	None	0.1	150	None

Continued

Table 7-10. PICU Large Volume Infusion Device and Syringe Pump Continuous Infusion Dosing Limits[6, 13–17] (cont'd)

Medication	Infusion Mode	Low Hard Limit	Low Soft Limit	High Soft Limit	High Hard Limit
Cyclosporine drip 1 mg/mL[b]	mg/hr	None	0.4	10	18
Cyclosporine intermittent dose ___mg/___mL	mL/hr	None	None	75	125
Dexmedetomidine drip 0.004 mg/mL	mcg/kg/hr	None	0.1	0.75	0.8
Diltiazem drip 1 mg/mL	mg/hr	None	5	None	15
Dobutamine drip (max) 5 mg/mL	mcg/kg/min	None	5	20	40
Dobutamine drip (std) 2 mg/mL	mcg/kg/min	None	5	20	40
Dopamine drip (double) 3.2 mg/mL	mcg/kg/min	None	5	20	50
Dopamine drip (max) 6.4 mg/mL	mcg/kg/min	None	5	20	50
Dopamine drip (std) 1.6 mg/mL	mcg/kg/min	None	5	20	50
Epinephrine drip (double) 0.04 mg/mL	mcg/kg/min	None	0.01	0.5	1
Epinephrine drip (max) 0.0064 mg/mL	mcg/kg/min	None	0.01	0.5	1
Epinephrine drip (std) 0.02 mg/mL	mcg/kg/min	None	0.01	0.5	1
Esmolol drip 20 mg/mL	mcg/kg/min	None	100	600	1000
Fosphenytoin dose ___mg/___mL	mL/hr	None	None	None	150
Furosemide drip 1 mg/mL	mg/kg/hr	None	0.05	0.6[c]	0.9[d]
Heparin drip 100 units/mL	units/kg/hr	None	10	30	99[e]
Immune globulin – sucrose ___g/___mL	mL/hr	None	None	None	150
Immune globulin – sucrose free ___g/___mL	mL/hr	None	None	None	250
Isoproterenol drip 20 mcg/mL	mcg/kg/min	None	0.05	1	2
IV fluid	mL/hr	None	0.1	150	None
IV fluid + KCl	mL/hr	None	0.1	150	300
K cocktail adult	mL/hr	None	25	50	99
K cocktail pediatric	mL/kg/hr	None	1	2	4
K/Na phosphorous replacement	mL/hr	None	0.1	None	55
Ketamine drip 2 mg/mL	mcg/kg/min	None	5	20	30[e]
Labetalol drip 5 mg/mL	mg/kg/hr	None	0.25	1	3
Lepirudin drip 0.4 mg/mL[a]	mg/kg/hr	None	None	0.15	None

Continued

Table 7-10. PICU Large Volume Infusion Device and Syringe Pump Continuous Infusion Dosing Limits[6, 13–17] (cont'd)

Medication	Infusion Mode	Low Hard Limit	Low Soft Limit	High Soft Limit	High Hard Limit
Lidocaine drip 8 mg/mL	mcg/kg/min	None	20	None	50
Lipid 20% (200 mg/mL)	mL/hr	0.1	1	25	50
Lorazepam drip 1 mg/mL[a]	mg/hr	None	0.01	0.09	0.1
Magnesium sulfate replacement 100 mg/mL	mL/hr	None	0.1	55	None
Midazolam drip 1 mg/mL	mg/kg/hr	None	0.03	0.2	0.4
Milrinone drip 0.2 mg/mL	mcg/kg/min	None	0.25	None	0.75
Mycophenolate 1000 mg/__mL	mL/hr	None	None	None	500
Mycophenolate 1500 mg/__mL	mL/hr	None	None	None	750
Naloxone drip 40 mcg/mL	mcg/kg/hr	None	0.25	3	160
Nesiritide drip 0.006 mg/mL[a]	mcg/kg/min	None	0.01	None	0.03
Nicardipine drip 0.1 mg/mL	mcg/kg/min	None	0.5	2.5	5.5
Nicardipine drip 0.4 mg/mL	mg/hr	None	0.5	2.5	5.5
Nitroglycerin drip 0.2 mg/mL	mcg/kg/min	None	0.25	5	20
Nitroprusside drip (max) 1.6 mg/mL + 16 mg/mL Na thiosulfate	mcg/kg/min	None	0.3	4	10
Nitroprusside drip (std) 0.4 mg/mL + 4 mg/mL Na thiosulfate	mcg/kg/min	None	0.3	4	10
Norepinephrine drip (max) 0.064 mg/mL	mcg/kg/min	None	0.05	0.5	2
Norepinephrine drip (std) 0.032 mg/mL	mcg/kg/min	None	0.05	0.5	2
Octreotide drip 5 mcg/mL	mcg/kg/hr	None	0.3	10	40
Ondansetron drip 1 mg/mL	mg/hr	None	0.5	None	1
Other drug	mL/hr	None	None	None	None
Pantoprazole drip 0.8 mg/mL[a]	mg/hr	None	None	None	8
Pentobarbital 8 mg/mL	mg/kg/hr	None	1	None	3
Phenylephrine drip 0.2 mg/mL	mcg/kg/min	None	0.1	0.5	3
Potassium chloride replacement 0.1 mEq/mL	mL/hr	None	0.1	225	275
Potassium chloride replacement 0.4 mEq/mL	mL/hr	None	0.1	55	70
Procainamide 8 mg/mL	mcg/kg/min	None	20	None	80
Propofol drip 100 mg/mL	mcg/kg/min	None	1	200	300
Ranitidine drip 1 mg/mL	mg/kg/hr	None	0.04	None	0.17
Sodium bicarbonate drip 1 mEq/mL	mEq/kg/hr	None	0.5	2	None
Tacrolimus drip 20 mcg/mL	mcg/hr	None	10	140	280

Continued

Table 7-10. PICU Large Volume Infusion Device and Syringe Pump Continuous Infusion Dosing Limits[6, 13–17] (cont'd)

Medication	Infusion Mode	Low Hard Limit	Low Soft Limit	High Soft Limit	High Hard Limit
Theophylline drip 1.6 mg/mL	mg/kg/hr	None	0.5	1.2	1.5
Thymoglobulin dose ___mg/___mL	mL/hr	None	None	70	None
TPN	mL/hr	None	0.1	150	None
Vancomycin ___mg/___mL	mL/hr	None	None	250	None
Vancomycin 1000 mg/250 mL	mL/hr	None	None	250	None
Vancomycin 1250 mg/250 mL	mL/hr	None	None	167	None
Vancomycin 500 mg/100 mL	mL/hr	None	None	100	None
Vancomycin 750 mg/150 mL	mL/hr	None	None	150	None
Vasopressin drip 1 unit/mL	units/kg/min	None	0.0003	None	0.01
Vecuronium drip 1 mg/mL	mcg/kg/min	None	1	None	2.5

[a]Extrapolated from adult dosing guidelines.

[b]Extrapolated from intermittent and/or maximum daily dosing information.

[c]Extrapolated from Bumex dosing.

[d]Extrapolated from adult dose of 40 mg/hr.

[e]High hard limit was raised due to clinical experience at our institution with ECMO patients requiring higher doses to achieve appropriate ACTs.

[f]High hard limit was raised to allow for titration in complex, tolerant patients.

Table 7-11. Syringe Pump Weight-Based Dosing Limits For Intermittent Infusions[6,7]

Medication	Low Hard Limit	Low Soft Limit	High Soft Limit	High Hard Limit
Abelcet	0.5 mg/kg	2.3 mg/kg	5.5 mg/kg	6 mg/kg
Acetazolamide	1 mg/kg	4.5 mg/kg	11 mg/kg	12 mg/kg
Acetylcysteine	7 mg/kg	63 mg/kg	77 mg/kg	165 mg/kg
Acyclovir	1 mg/kg	4.5 mg/kg	22 mg/kg	24 mg/kg
Albumin	0.1 g/kg	0.23 g/kg	1.1. g/kg	1.2 g/kg
Amikacin	1 mg/kg	4.5 mg/kg	22 mg/kg	33 mg/kg
Aminophylline	0.25 mg/kg	0.9 mg/kg	2.75 mg/kg	3 mg/kg
Amphotericin B	0.1 mg/kg	0.23 mg/kg	1.65 mg/kg	1.8 mg/kg
Ampicillin	10 mg/kg	22 mg/kg	110 mg/kg	120 mg/kg
Ampicillin/sulbactam	10 mg/kg	22 mg/kg	165 mg/kg	180 mg/kg
Anti-thrombin III	6 units/kg	36 units/kg	66 units/kg	None
Azathioprine	0.5 mg/kg	0.9 mg/kg	5.5 mg/kg	6 mg/kg
Azithromycin	1 mg/kg	4.5 mg/kg	11 mg/kg	12 mg/kg
Aztreonam	5 mg/kg	27 mg/kg	55 mg/kg	77 mg/kg
Bumetanide	0.005 mg/kg	0.013 mg/kg	0.11 mg/kg	0.15 mg/kg

Continued

Table 7-11. Syringe Pump Weight-Based Dosing Limits For Intermittent Infusions[6,7] (cont'd)

Medication	Low Hard Limit	Low Soft Limit	High Soft Limit	High Hard Limit
Caffeine citrate	0.5 mg/kg	4.5 mg/kg	22 mg/kg	24 mg/kg
Calcium chloride	2 mg/kg	9 mg/kg	22 mg/kg	24 mg/kg
Calcium gluconate	10 mg/kg	45 mg/kg	110 mg/kg	250 mg/kg
Carnitine	5 mg/kg	27 mg/kg	55 mg/kg	60 mg/kg
Caspofungin	7 mg/m^2	45 mg/m^2	77 mg/m^2	84 mg/m^2
Cefazolin	3 mg/kg	7 mg/kg	37 mg/kg	40 mg/kg
Cefepime	5 mg/kg	27 mg/kg	55 mg/kg	60 mg/kg
Cefotaxime	5 mg/kg	22 mg/kg	110 mg/kg	120 mg/kg
Cefoxitin	4 mg/kg	12 mg/kg	44 mg/kg	48 mg/kg
Ceftazidime	5 mg/kg	22 mg/kg	55 mg/kg	77 mg/kg
Ceftriaxone	10 mg/kg	22 mg/kg	110 mg/kg	120 mg/kg
Cefuroxime	5 mg/kg	22 mg/kg	86 mg/kg	96 mg/kg
Chloramphenicol	2.5 mg/kg	6 mg/kg	28 mg/kg	30 mg/kg
Chlorothiazide	0.1 mg/kg	0.8 mg/kg	9 mg/kg	22 mg/kg
Ciprofloxacin	1 mg/kg	4.5 mg/kg	16 mg/kg	18 mg/kg
Clindamycin	1 mg/kg	4.5 mg/kg	14 mg/kg	15.6 mg/kg
Desmopressin	0.03 mcg/kg	0.27 mcg/kg	0.33 mcg/kg	0.36 mcg/kg
Dexamethasone	0.05 mg/kg	0.22 mg/kg	0.66 mg/kg	2.1 mg/kg
Digoxin	0.2 mcg/kg	1.8 mcg/kg	6.6 mcg/kg	28 mcg/kg
Diltiazem	0.03 mg/kg	0.22 mg/kg	0.38 mg/kg	0.42 mg/kg
Diphenhydramine	0.1 mg/kg	0.45 mg/kg	2.2 mg/kg	2.4 mg/kg
Doxycycline	0.4 mg/k/g	1.8 mg/kg	4.4. mg/kg	4.8 mg/kg
Enalaprilat	0.5 mcg/kg	4.5 mcg/kg	27.5 mcg/kg	None
Epoetin alfa	2.5 units/kg	22.5 units/kg	330 units/kg	360 units/kg
Erythromycin lactobionate	0.4 mg/kg	3 mg/kg	5.5 mg/kg	13.8 mg/kg
Fentanyl	None	0.45 mcg/kg	2.2 mcg/kg	25 mcg/kg
Filgrastim	1 mcg/kg	4.5 mcg/kg	11 mcg/kg	12 mcg/kg
Fluconazole	0.3 mg/kg	1.3 mg/kg	13 mg/kg	14.4 mg/kg
Foscarnet	6 mg/kg	16 mg/kg	66 mg/kg	132 mg/kg
Fosphenytoin	2 mg/kg	9 mg/kg	22 mg/kg	24 mg/kg
Furosemide	0.1 mg/kg	0.45 mg/kg	2.2 mg/kg	6.6 mg/kg
Ganciclovir	0.5 mg/kg	0.56 mg/kg	5.5 mg/kg	6.6 mg/kg
Gentamicin	0.1 mg/kg	0.9 mg/kg	11 mg/kg	16.5 mg/kg
Glycopyrrolate	1 mcg/kg	3.6 mcg/kg	11 mcg/kg	12 mcg/kg
Granisetron	4 mcg/kg	9 mcg/kg	44 mcg/kg	48 mcg/kg
Hydralazine	0.02 mg/kg	0.09 mg/kg	0.55 mg/kg	0.88 mg/kg
Hydrocortisone	0.05 mg/kg	0.45 mg/kg	2.75 mg/kg	55 mg/kg
Hydromorphone	None	0.005 mg/kg	0.033 mg/kg	0.11 mg/kg

Continued

Table 7-11. Syringe Pump Weight-Based Dosing Limits For Intermittent Infusions[6,7] (cont'd)

Medication	Low Hard Limit	Low Soft Limit	High Soft Limit	High Hard Limit
Hydroxyzine	0.1 mg/kg	0.45 mg/kg	1.1 mg/kg	1.2 mg/kg
Imipenem/cilastin	2.5 mg/kg	13.5 mg/kg	27.5 mg/kg	55 mg/kg
Indomethacin	0.025 mg/kg	0.09 mg/kg	0.275 mg/kg	0.3 mg/kg
Ketorolac	0.05 mg/kg	0.45 mg/kg	0.55 mg/kg	1.1 mg/kg
Labetalol	0.05 mg/kg	0.18 mg/kg	0.55 mg/kg	1.1 mg/kg
Leucovorin	1 mg/m²	9 mg/m²	11 mg/m²	13.2 mg/m²
Levofloxacin	1 mg/kg	2.2 mg/kg	11 mg/kg	12 mg/kg
Levothyroxine	0.75 mcg/kg	1.8 mcg/kg	8.3 mcg/kg	12 mcg/kg
Linezolid	1 mg/kg	9 mg/kg	11 mg/kg	12 mg/kg
Meropenem	4 mg/kg	9 mg/kg	44 mg/kg	55 mg/kg
Magnesium sulfate	5 mg/kg	22.5 mg/kg	55 mg/kg	110 mg/kg
Methadone	None	0.009 mg/kg	0.22 mg/kg	0.55 mg/kg
Methylprednisolone	0.05 mg/kg	0.23 m/gkg	16.5 mg/kg	33 mg/kg
Metoclopramide	0.02 mg/kg	0.09 mg/kg	0.22 mg/kg	2.2 mg/kg
Metronidazole	1.5 mg/kg	6.8 mg/kg	16.5 mg/kg	18 mg/kg
Midazolam	None	0.009 mg/kg	0.22 mg/kg	0.55 mg/kg
Morphine	None	0.009 mg/kg	0.22 mg/kg	0.55 mg/kg
Mycophenolate	60 mg/m²	270 mg/m²	660 mg/m²	720 mg/m²
Nafcillin	5 mg/kg	22.5 mg/kg	55 mg/kg	60 mg/kg
Octreotide	0.1 mcg/kg	0.9 mcg/kg	11 mcg/kg	12 mcg/kg
Ondansetron	0.02 mg/kg	0.09 mg/kg	0.22 mg/kg	0.24 mg/kg
Pantoprazole	0.1 mg/kg	0.45 mg/kg	1.1 mg/kg	2.2 mg/kg
Phenobarbital	0.2 mg/kg	0.9 mg/kg	22 mg/kg	33 mg/kg
Phytonadione	0.1 mg	1 mg	10 mg	20 mg
Piperacillin	7.5 mg/kg	22.5 mg/kg	83 mg/kg	110 mg/kg
Piperacillin/tazobactam	8 mg/kg	54 mg/kg	110 mg/kg	120 mg/kg
Potassium chloride	0.05 mEq/kg	0.225 mEq/kg	0.55 mEq/kg	1.1 mEq/kg
Prochlorperazine	0.015 mg/kg	0.09 mg/kg	0.165 mg/kg	0.18 mg/kg
Promethazine	0.1 mg/kg	0.22 mg/kg	1.1 mg/kg	1.2 mg/kg
Propranolol	0.001 mg/kg	0.009 mg/kg	0.275 mg/kg	0.3 mg/kg
Quinupristin/dalfopristin	0.75 mg/kg	6.75 mg/kg	8.25 mg/kg	9 mg/kg
Ranitidine	0.05 mg/kg	0.1 mg/kg	1.65 mg/kg	1.8 mg/kg
Rifampin	2 mg/kg	4.5 mg/kg	22 mg/kg	24 mg/kg
Sodium bicarbonate	0.1 mEq/kg	0.45 mEq/kg	2.2 mEq/kg	2.4 mEq/kg
Ticarcillin/clavulanate	10 mg/kg	45 mg/kg	110 mg/kg	120 mg/kg
Tobramycin	0.1 mg/kg	0.9 mg/kg	11 mg/kg	16.5 mg/kg
TMP/sulfamethoxazole	0.2 mg/kg	1.8 mg/kg	11 mg/kg	12 mg/kg
Tromethamine	None	None	500 mL	None

Continued

Table 7-11. Syringe Pump Weight-Based Dosing Limits For Intermittent Infusions[6,7] [cont'd]

Medication	Low Hard Limit	Low Soft Limit	High Soft Limit	High Hard Limit
Valproate	1 mg/kg	2.25 mg/kg	44 mg/kg	48 mg/kg
Vancomycin	1.5 mg/kg	9 mg/kg	22 mg/kg	30 mg/kg
Voriconazole	0.8 mg/kg	2.7 mg/kg	8.8 mg/kg	12 mg/kg
Zidovudine	0.15 mg/kg	1.35 mg/kg	1.65 mg/kg	1.8 mg/kg

Table 7-12. PICU Large Volume Infusion Device Non-Weight-Based Bolus Dosing Limits [< 45 Kg][6,7]

Medication for Bolus Dose	Low Hard Limit	Low Soft Limit	High Soft Limit	High Hard Limit
IV fluid	None	50 mL	1000 mL	None
Aminophylline	None	10 mg	270 mg	300 mg
Aminocaproic acid	None	500 mg	4500 mg	5000 mg
Amiodarone	None	25 mg	225 mg	250 mg
Bumetanide	None	0.07 mg	0.7 mg	1 mg
Calcium chloride	None	50 mg	1000 mg	1500 mg
Calcium gluconate	None	200 mg	2000 mg	3000 mg
Cisatracurium	None	0.5 mg	4.5 mg	9 mg
Dexmedetomidine	None	2.5 mcg	45 mcg	50 mcg
Diltiazem	None	1.25 mg	16 mg	20 mg
Esmolol	None	500 mcg	22,500 mcg	25,000 mcg
Heparin	None	100 units	2250 units	2500 units
Labetalol	None	1 mg	45 mg	50 mg
Lepirudin	None	1 mg	20 mg	25 mg
Lidocaine	None	5 mg	45 mg	50 mg
Milrinone	None	250 mcg	2250 mcg	2500 mcg
Nesiritide	None	5 mcg	90 mg	100 mcg
Octreotide	None	5 mcg	45 mcg	50 mcg
Propofol	None	5 mg	160 mg	200 mg
Theophylline	None	10 mg	270 mg	300 mg

Table 7-13. PICU Large Volume Infusion Device Weight-Based Bolus Dosing Limits[6,7]

Medication for Bolus Dose	Low Hard Limit	Low Soft Limit	High Soft Limit	High Hard Limit
IV fluid	None	10 mL/kg	15 mL/kg	None
Aminophylline	None	5 mg/kg	6 mg/kg	6.6 mg/kg
Aminocaproic acid	None	75 mg/kg	100 mg/kg	110 mg/kg
Amiodarone	None	3.75 mg/kg	5 mg/kg	5.5 mg/kg
Bumetanide	None	0.01 mg/kg	0.015 mg/kg	0.17 mg/kg
Calcium chloride	None	10 mg/kg	20 mg/kg	22 mg/kg
Calcium gluconate	None	40 mg/kg	100 mg/kg	110 mg/kg
Cisatracurium	None	0.05 mg/kg	0.1 mg/kg	0.2 mg/kg
Dexmedetomidine	None	0.5 mcg/kg	1 mcg/kg	1.1 mcg/kg
Diltiazem	None	0.25 mg/kg	0.35 mg/kg	0.4 mg/kg
Esmolol	None	100 mcg/kg	500 mcg/kg	550 mcg/kg
Heparin	None	25 units/kg	50 units/kg	60 units/kg
Labetalol	None	0.2 mg/kg	1 mg/kg	1.1 mg/kg
Lepirudin	None	0.2 mg/kg	0.4 mg/kg	0.45 mg/kg
Lidocaine	None	0.75 mg/kg	1 mg/kg	1.5 mg/kg
Milrinone	None	25 mcg/kg	50 mcg/kg	55 mcg/kg
Nesiritide	None	1 mcg/kg	2 mcg/kg	2.2 mcg/kg
Octreotide	None	0.75 mcg/kg	1 mcg/kg	1.1 mcg/kg
Propofol	None	1.5 mg/kg	3.5 mg/kg	3.9 mg/kg
Theophylline	None	5 mg/kg	6 mg/kg	6.6 mg/kg

PRACTICE TIPS

Borrowing a Library

- Infusion pump libraries from other institutions can be an invaluable resource when developing your own set of pediatric libraries.
- Borrowed libraries should be closely reviewed to ensure that the medication entries are set up according to your preferred naming conventions, standard concentrations, and standard volumes.
- Dosing limits should also be thoroughly reviewed to make sure they agree with policies and practice at your site.

Use of Special Alerts

- Some software allows special alerts to be placed within drug entries. Examples of alerts that could be added are "Central Line Only," "High-Alert Medication: Requires a Double-Check," or "Caution: Cytotoxic."
- When used appropriately, these alerts can be valuable tools for the pediatric nurse to ensure safe administration or handling of a drug.

- Caution should be taken to carefully plan use of these alerts, as too many could lead to alert fatigue.

Multiple Types of Pumps with Differing Drug Libraries

- When multiple types of pumps with potentially different libraries are in use in a pediatric area, there should be clear guidelines for when to use each type of pump, library, and/or library entry.
- Medication labels, electronic medication orders, and flow-sheet nomenclature can sometimes be valuable tools to ensure correct pump/library choices are made.
- Whenever possible, drug name, concentration, and units on medication labels and flow-sheets should exactly match what the nurse is looking for in the pump library.
- Upon order entry, we found that using weight cut-off descriptors helped our prescribers choose the correct infusion entry for the patient, which in turn mapped to the correct concentration, volume, and container type (syringe vs. bag). For instance in our computerized provider order entry system, we have a choice for "Midazolam Drip – Peds < 45 kg" and "Midazolam Drip – Adult." The pediatric entry maps to a syringe and the adult entry maps to a bag for dispensing. The type of container dispensed then leads the nurse to the correct pump choice.

Bolus Infusion Programming Units

- Whenever possible, choose bolus dose units that agree with how bolus doses are ordered at your site. Nurses should not be expected to perform calculations in order to program a bolus dose into an infusion device.
- If the software will not allow the choice you desire, consider changing ordering practices or utilizing other technology to prevent hand-calculations.
- When the syringe pump at our site would only allow weight-based bolus dose programming (because we had selected a weight-based mode of infusion delivery), we were able to utilize out CPOE system to automatically calculate a mcg/kg dose conversion for affected medications. For instance, if a physician orders 10 mcg of fentanyl on a 10 kg patient, the computer system automatically calculates that the dose is 1 mcg/kg for bolus doses given through a syringe pump and displays this on the electronic medication administration record.

Patient Weight Changes

- Develop a plan for how to handle changes in patient weight, as infants and children may grow significantly during a hospital stay.

- Our interdisciplinary teams agree upon a dosing weight for medications, rather than using the daily weight. The dosing weight is updated in the computer system during medical rounds only when the team feels that a significant amount of weight change has occurred. Medication infusions and pump programming are adjusted at that time.

Library Validation Process

- Schedule a library validation session prior to implementation. Involve representatives from the pediatric nursing, pediatric pharmacy, and bio-medical electronics departments at a minimum.
- Load the library onto a test pump.
- Verify that the library functions on the pump as intended and that all of the line item entries are correct.
- Run through several common patient scenarios, to ensure that your library design is workable and problem-free.
- When possible, include bedside nurses in the validation process to lend real-life expertise.

Effecting Practice Change

- Pediatrics is a high-risk group for medication errors. Share with all inter-disciplinary team members the compelling reasons behind implementation of intelligent infusion device technology early in the process to create a shared vision for change.
- If possible, share site specific data about adverse events or errors that may have been prevented by smart pump technology.
- Include interdisciplinary team members in all steps of the decision and review processes and identify key individuals to act as change agents.
- Provide easily accessible information, such as dosing cheat cards, for pump library changes necessitating a change in physician ordering practices.

References

1. Larsen GY, Parker HB, Cash J, O'Connell M, Grant MC. Standard drug concentrations and smart-pump technology reduce continuous-medication-infusion errors in pediatric patients. *Pediatrics.* 2005;116:e21-e25.

2. Lesar T. Errors in the use of medication dosage equations. *Arch Pediatr Adolesc Med.* 1998; 152:340-344.

3. Kaushal R. Medication errors and adverse drug events in pediatric inpatients. *JAMA.* 2001;286:915-916.

4. Vanderveen T. Smart pumps: advanced capabilities and continuous quality improvement. *Patient Saf Qual Healthcare.* Jan/Feb 2007;1-13.

5. Proceedings from the ISMP summit on the use of smart infusion pumps: guidelines for safe implementation and use. Available at: www.ismp.org. Accessed October 14, 2009.

6. Taketomo CK, Hodding JH, Kraus DM. *Pediatric Dosage Handbook*. 14th ed. Hudson, OH: Lexi-Comp, Inc; 2007.

7. Lacy CF, Armstrong LL, Goldman MP, Lance LL. *Drug Information Handbook*. 17th ed. Hudson, OH: Lexi-Comp, Inc; 2008.

8. Trissel LA. *Handbook on Injectable Drugs*. 15th ed. Bethesda, MD: American Society of Health-System Pharmacists, Inc; 2008.

9. Phelps SJ, Hak EB, Crill CM. *Pediatric Injectable Drugs*. 8th ed. Bethesda, MD: American Society of Health-System Pharmacists, Inc; 2007.

10. Gahart BL, Nazareno AR. 2009 *Intravenous Medications*. St. Louis, MO: Mosby Inc; 2009.

11. Bing CM. *Extended Stability of Parenteral Drugs*. 3rd ed. Bethesda, MD: American Society of Health-System Pharmacists, Inc; 2005.

12. McEvoy GK, ed. AHFS Drug Information 2008. Bethesda, MD: American Society of Health-System Pharmacists, Inc; 2008.

13. Refludan (lepirudin [rDNA]) IV injection (package insert). Wayne, NJ: Bayer Healthcare; 2006.

14. Jacobi J, Fraser GL, Coursin DB, et al. Clinical practice guidelines for the sustained use of sedatives and analgesics in the critically ill adult. *Crit Care Med*. 2002;30(1):119-141.

15. Natrecor (nesiritide) IV injection (package insert). Fremont, CA: Scios, Inc.; 2005.

16. Huggins RM, Scates AC, Latour JK. Intravenous proton-pump inhibitors versus H2-antagonists for treatment of GI bleeding. *Ann Pharmacother*. 37(3):433-437.

17. Mortimer DS, Jancik J. Administering hypertonic saline to patients with severe traumatic brain injury. *J Neurosci Nurs*. 38(3):142-146.

Building Drug Library Subsets

Pamela K. Phelps and Michelle L. Borchart

Key Terms

Drug library subsets—a subset of the larger drug library that includes all drugs needed for a specific patient population or area. Other names that pump vendors use for these subsets are personalities, profiles, and clinical care areas.

High "hard" dose limit—a high dose limit programmed into a pump; the pump cannot be programmed higher than a high "hard" limit. The user must use a dose lower than this limit.

Nesting—grouping varying drug concentrations under a single drug name. This avoids having both concentrations show up on the main screen, thereby avoiding excessive scrolling.

Scrolling—reading through drug names on the pump in order to find the desired drug name. If a drug list is fairly long, excessive scrolling can be inefficient.

Introduction: Division of the Drug Library

After building your health system's drug library, you will find that it will be very large and difficult to navigate. This is where dividing the drug library into smaller, easier to navigate lists known as drug library subsets, clinical care areas, profiles or personalities will help with ease of use. Dividing a smart pump drug library into drug library subsets could be compared to separating an mp3 player's general music library into separate playlists.

Steps in Building Drug Library Subsets

Choosing Number and Names of Drug Library Subsets

The first step in developing drug library subsets is deciding how many your institution/health system is going to have and what they will be. It is important to find out how many your chosen pump will allow in its software. The number of drug library subsets allowed varies significantly for different smart pumps on the market. Some only hold approximately 10; others can hold 40 or more. To decide number of drug library subsets needed, your pump development group will have to decide the method by which they will divide out the drug library subsets. Choices of how to divide the drug library subsets include by patient populations, patient care areas of the hospital, patient weights, and individual hospitals, if implementing smart pumps for a health system. Drug library subsets can be chosen based on a variety of patient characteristics. For example, you may want individual drug libraries set up for different geographic areas or patient care areas of the hospital. Conversely, pediatric drug library subsets may be organized by patient weight, without regard for the location of the patient.

Typical drug library subsets identified by health systems and hospitals include Emergency Department, Med/Surg, Labor and Delivery, Obstetrics/Gynecology, Pediatrics, Pediatric ICU, Neonatal ICU, Adult Critical Care, Renal Services/ Dialysis, Anesthesiology, Cardiac Catheterization and Chemotherapy/Biologics.[1] A drug library subset for a Code Team can be built with wider dose limits or an absence of dose limits. It is common to break pediatric drug libraries up by patient weight in order to minimize the number of different drug concentrations in each drug library subset. Weight based drug library subsets also allow the programmer to set tighter limits, thus improving patient safety for high-risk drugs used in pediatric patients.[2] Examples of drug library subsets are listed in Table 8-1.

In implementing intelligent pumps for a health system, it may be necessary to have separate drug library subsets for each separate hospital. If one of the hospitals has a unique patient population (transplant patients, for example) and the other hospitals do not, it may be beneficial to have a drug library subset of transplant medications for just that hospital. Likewise, if the health system has some large hospitals and some smaller hospitals, it may be beneficial for the smaller hospitals to have their own drug library subset in order to customize for their own needs.

Table 8-1. Drug Library Subset Examples

Drug Library Subset Names	Service Line	Description
University ICU	ICU-general	Critical care at teaching Hospital
ICU	ICU-general	Critical care at non-teaching institutions
OB	Obstetrics/gynecology	
Peds-gen	Medicine-pediatrics	Pediatrics 5–45 kg
PICU	ICU-pediatrics	ICU pediatrics 5–45 kg
ICU 0–5 kg	ICU-neonatal	Infants <5 kg in NICU and PICU
0–5 kg	Medicine-pediatric	Infants <5 kg
Med surg	Medicine-adult	
Chem/bio	Oncology-adult	Oncology and bone marrow transplant

Creating new drug library subsets for smaller hospitals or unique patient populations may allow for a shorter list of medications in each drug library subset.[1] Having fewer medications in each drug library subset gives the nurse fewer medications and medication concentrations to choose from, thereby decreasing the likelihood of choosing the wrong medication or medication concentration.

It may also be beneficial to include a test library. This is especially useful during the development stages of the drug library. A test library may allow for testing of certain medication settings on the pump. This library can also be used for training purposes for end users of the pump. For reporting purposes, the test library can be excluded from the data. One risk of having a test library is that it may be used by pump users by mistake. This can be prevented in some pumps be password protecting the library so only those who know the password can access the library. It is beneficial to include a test library.

Drug Library Subset Congruence with Guiding Principles

When beginning to organize medications from the general drug library into separate drug library subsets, it is important for the health system to go back and look at their guiding principles for pump implementation. Some hospitals/health systems will elect to make their drug library subsets very broad in nature. This will lessen the need for searching to find a drug library subset, but will increase the need for scrolling to find the medication. A broader drug library subset will require a larger number of medications in that subset. Broader drug libraries offer the advantage of nurses being more likely able to use one drug library subset for the majority of their patients. Requiring a nurse to go outside of their usual drug library subset can be time consuming in some pump models, but in other pumps can be very easy. Other hospitals/health systems may elect to create narrower drug library subsets, with a drug library subset for each nursing unit. Narrower drug libraries will minimize the amount of scrolling time to find medications, but this will increase the need for nurses to practice in multiple drug library subsets as they travel to different care units. In this case, using a dual-channel pump with the ability to use separate library subsets for each channel could be a good solution.

Adding Medications to Drug Library Subsets

After decisions have been made as to the amount, type, and breadth of the drug library subsets, you can begin to build the drug library subsets. If your drug library subsets are organized by patient care areas or nursing units, it is essential to start with either a computer-generated report of utilization, or simply asking someone who works in that area to make a list of the most commonly used IV medications. Typically, the pharmacy department owns the building of the drug library, and the actual software programming. A pharmacist will build basic drug library subsets and then bring together groups of professionals to provide feedback on additions and deletions to their drug library subset. By and large, decisions regarding which drugs go into which clinical care area should be driven by utilization patterns and nursing preference.

Arrangement of Medications in Drug Library Subsets

Organization of medications in the drug library subsets is very important for ease of use. A common way to organize the medications is to place the most commonly used medications at the top of the list. This will place these drugs on the first few display screens after the drug library subset is chosen by a bedside caregiver. Medications frequently placed at the top of the list include IV fluids, blood products, electrolyte replacements, a generic antibiotic line item, TPN (total parenteral nutrition), and lipids. After listing the most frequently used medications and fluids, the rest of the medications in the drug display can be listed out in alphabetical order. The organization of medications for drug display in drug library subsets is another area where nursing input is essential. Nursing should generate a list for each area of the medications they would like to see displayed at the top of the list, as well as how they would like to see the remainder of the list displayed.

Some brands of pumps will only allow medications to be arranged in alphabetical order. When using pumps that require medications to be displayed in alphabetical order in drug library subsets it requires more careful thought in naming medications. One option for isolating out certain medications such as chemotherapy in a drug library subset that only allows arrangement by alphabetical order is to label the medications with a "z" before the name. A example of this would be listing chemotherapy medications as z-amifostine and z-arsenic trioxide. This would allow chemotherapy to be listed in the same drug library subset as other medications, but be separated out.

Nesting of Drug Names

Another topic to discuss regarding the display of medications in drug library subsets is the "nesting" of drug names. It is important to discover if this feature is available for your chosen pump. Let's say you have multiple concentrations of dopamine infusion. If nesting is used and dopamine is selected on the pump screen, various concentrations of dopamine can be "nested" under the parent name, dopamine. As such, a nurse can choose "dopamine," and then make the decision of which dopamine concentration should be used (for example 800 mg/250 mL). All available concentrations of the selected drug will then appear under the parent name of that drug. In order for "nesting" to be available on the pump, all concentrations of a given drug have to be programmed with the exact same displayed name. If your health system has standard dosages for IV medications, these also may be nested. See Figure 8-1.

Transfer of Patients

Transfer procedures for patients leaving one nursing unit and going to another should be considered. Policies regarding the need to change drug library subsets upon transfer should be developed.[2] The health system should make a decision whether the receiving nurse will need to stop and re-program the pump, using their usual drug library subset, work outside of their usual drug library subset upon transfer until a new bag is hung, or continue to work outside of their usual drug library subset until the infusion is discontinued. Multiple channel pumps will allow the nurse to use different drug library subsets for the different channels.

Review of Drug Library Subsets

An essential part of the creation of drug library subsets is the review process. Once each subset has been created it is important to review the subset with a group of nurses who will be using that drug library subset a majority of the time. To save time, send out a list of the medications with dose limits in the drug library subset to the group in advance, so they can look at the list before meeting face-to-face. Then bring a pump with the medication subset loaded onto the pump, so that the bedside caregivers can see how the limits actually function on the pump. This will help the bedsides caregivers begin to familiarize themselves with the pump. Ask the group for suggestions of how they would like to see the drug library subset changed; would they like to add any medications, would they

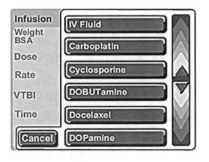
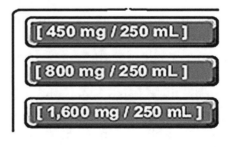

Figure 8-1. Examples of nesting. *Source:* Printed with permission of Hospira.

like to remove any medications, or would they like to reorganize the list. After the drug library subset review send out the updated list and again ask for suggestions for changes. The drug library subset review process may be a lengthy process and require many revisions, but it is important to have good drug library subset before pump "go live." The more satisfied your pump users are with the arrangement and contents of the drug library, subset the more likely they will be to utilize the drug libraries for their infusions.

Drug library subsets should be reviewed and evaluated post-implementation for user satisfaction. The amount and type of drug library subsets should be evaluated, as well as the arrangement of medications in the subsets. This could be done by nursing surveys, as well as by reports generated by the pump software. The software will help to determine compliance with use of drug libraries. It may be necessary to reorganize medications in the drug library subsets or build new drug library subsets a few months post-implementation, if user compliance with the drug libraries is poor. The software reports are covered in depth in a future chapter. Keep in mind that development and maintenance of drug library subsets is a dynamic process. It will need to be evaluated and resourced after pump implementation.

Final Approval of the Drug Library

The pump implementation committee will require final approval of the drug library before the smart pump goes live at any institution. The drug library sign-off can come from an individual involved in pump software programming or from a designated hospital committee. One likely approval body is the pharmacy and therapeutics committee. the pharmacy and therapeutics committee can quickly review the library and look for any major issues after review by nursing and pharmacy. The value of pharmacy and therapeutics committee approval is in the endorsement of the library by the committee. Endorsement by the pharmacy and therapeutics committee will aid in ensuring compliance with the safety features of the pump.

Conclusion

Drug library subsets should allow your pump users to navigate the smart pump drug library with greater ease. The drug library subsets are a balance between safety and convenience. The drug list should allow users to find the medications that they need, yet be complete enough to take advantage of the safety software embedded in the pump. The way medications are organized within the drug library subset will have a large impact on the pump user. Nursing should determine their preferences on how they would like to see medications ordered within the drug library subsets. Multiple disciplines can aid in the drug library review process by making suggestions for fine-tuning the drug library subsets, and checking limits for accuracy. The more time that is spent reviewing and gaining user input on drug library subsets before pump implementation, the more likely pump users will be utilize the pump libraries for programming infusions. You should also reinforce the idea that pump programming is a dynamic process; if utilization reports indicate that a medication is not used in a particular area, it can be removed from the subset. Continuing to refine the medication lists and subsets will aid in user satisfaction over the long run.

PRACTICE TIPS

- Develop a list of potential library subsets. Recognize that this will change during the process.
- Decide on a philosophy for nursing use of multiple library subsets. Will this be encouraged or discouraged?
- Run pharmacy reports to determine frequency of medication utilization in each area.
- Ask nurses to determine the ordering (rank) of medication in the library subset.
- Develop a patient transfer process that addresses whether or not the library subset will be changed after transfer.
- Nest drugs in the pump library, when possible.
- Keep in mind that it is a dynamic process; changes will be made based on user feedback and pump software reports.

References

1. Siv-Lee L, Morgan L. Implementation of Wireless "intelligent" pump IV infusion technology in a not-for-profit academic hospital setting. *Hosp Pharm.* 2007;42:832-840.
2. Cohen MR, Schneider P, Niemi K. Effective approaches to standardization and implementation of smart pump technology. *ISMP.* 2007.

Education for "Go-Live"

Burnis D. Breland

CHAPTER 9

Key Terms

Clinician compliance—the extent to which caregivers use the pump as was intended; programming the pump using the safety software.

Dose error reduction system (DERS)—term used to describe software built into intelligent infusion devices that is designed to catch dosing or administration errors. In this case, it represents the programming of minimum and maximum dose limits in an infusion pump, and the alerts presented to the clinician when programmed doses are exceeded.

Drug library—a comprehensive list of medications and fluids that are to be delivered using the infusion pump. This library includes any dose, volume, or rate limitations that are programmed into the software.

Go-live—the day that is chosen to switch from the current pump to the newer smart pump. On go-live day, old pumps must be exchanged for new pumps, or "swapped out." Nursing and pharmacy must collaborate to provide new tubing, new medication infusions, and to accurately re-program the new pump.

Safety software—see definition for DERS above.

Smart infusion pumps—a new generation of infusion pumps that incorporates dose limiting software into the pump hardware; this software is designed to prevent infusion-related programming errors. The Joint Commission, in the 2006 National Patient Safety Goals, defined a smart pump as a "parenteral infusion pump equipped with IV medication error-prevention software that alerts operators or interrupts the infusion process when a pump setting is programmed outside of pre-configured limits." Smart pumps are designed to recognize prescription errors, dose misinterpretations, and keypad programming errors.

Super-users—individuals involved in the selection and implementation of
   smart pumps who feel familiar enough with the processes to educate others.
   Super-users may be relied upon to mentor other users not as familiar with
   the technology. Super-users may also conduct formal training sessions.

Introduction

Educating clinicians before implementing intelligent infusion systems (smart
pumps) is essential to making a smooth transition from an older system. This
chapter will discuss the framework to developing an effective education plan for
the "go-live" day of your institution's intelligent infusion systems. Furthermore, it
will explain the creation of training modules and the evaluation and assessment
after the new system is in place.

Create the Education Plan

To successfully "go live" with new technology, such as an intelligent infusion system
with safety software, a thorough education plan is imperative. Only when nurses
are comfortable and secure in their use of the new technology will their compliance and use of the safety software be optimal. Clinician compliance is essential
to help optimize and take full advantage of the new intelligent infusion system.

Keep in mind that change is intimidating for many people, so a positive,
upbeat attitude is important in relaying information about the new technology.
Reinforce also that the new system supports nurses, and does not diminish the
important work they do every day. An intelligent infusion system is designed to
prevent medication errors or miscalculations, but will still rely on nurses' professional sensibilities/critical thinking and judgment when providing treatment for
their patients.

Developing the education plan should begin as soon as it is clear that an
intelligent infusion system will be installed in your hospital. Steps include:

Step 1: Define the education team. Usually the education team, made up of
pharmacists, nurses, nurse educators and/or nurse administrators, risk management specialists and biomedical personnel will take on the task of nurse
and pharmacist education in addition to the drug library development.
There are at least three members on a team, but there may be more for larger institutions. From this team, a leader should be identified to oversee the
implementation plans and execution of the education plan. The team leader
should be knowledgeable regarding infusion system issues and be detail
and results-oriented. Most of all, the project leader must be interested and
committed to successful project implementation. A pharmacist or nurse may
either serve as an effective leader. The number of personnel on the team
depends on your institution's needs—a pharmacist, two nurses and a team

leader may be enough for smaller institutions; larger institutions may require more. Remember that, just as with the entire project team, adding new technology requires time and dedication from some of your most valued staff. The staff who know the processes the best are often front line staff and front line managers and pulling them away of patient care responsibilities or diverting a managers time may be disruptive. Therefore, they should be relieved of some of their regular duties or given support from other staff or managers while assisting in the process plan development and execution. If this is not possible then senior management will need to determine where resources can be obtained or redirected to provide the proper support.

Step 2: Develop a timeline. A timeline for nurse education should correspond with the timeline developed by the project team for the entire implementation process (product installation, policy and procedure assessment and standardization, drug library development, and time for hands-on testing). Adequate training will usually require multiple sessions so all nurses can attend. Be sure to provide enough lead time prior to the "go-live" target date to accommodate the number of nurses who will need to be educated, the frequency of the classes, and refresher classes if needed. Training schedules should be flexible to accommodate all shifts and must be mandatory so all clinicians are adequately trained. You don't want to reach "go-live" with many of your staff unprepared to use the new devices.

Generally, there is only one training session necessary per nurse with multiple sessions available to accommodate all staff. The training is instructive with take home materials and offers hands-on practice and opportunity for demonstration of competency. During the drug library build, there can be several sessions to review the drug library. This is required to ensure adequate training with hands on practice with the devices and allow for an understanding of the library. Each session may last up to 2 hours in length, dependent on the device. The sessions are usually limited to 10 nurses per class and must be done to accommodate both night and weekend staff. Also consider off site nurses and staff. Allow from 2 to 4 weeks or more for training, depending on the size of institution.

Step 3: Assess the number of people who will need to be educated. Everyone who will potentially administer an IV solution in your institution should receive education/training on the new safety software intelligent infusion pumps. Don't forget to include the anesthesiologists in the OR, perhaps physicians in the emergency department, and pharmacists. Education should be mandatory. Selective usage of the pumps by those unwilling to learn and use the technology will diminish the efficiency and cost-effectiveness of the technology.

Defining the number of personnel to be trained will help in deciding the size of the classes, scheduling enough classes within the normal work shift, finding adequate space and enough pumps for each training class, and identifying the number of super-users (see below) needed to support your program. You may want to stagger training by clinical care area or other convenient grouping to help minimize impact on day-to-day services. Training should be mandatory for all potential intelligent pump users.

Step 4: Create a team of "super-users." Super-users are individuals who exhibit special interest in using the new intelligent device system can be selected early in the implementation process and given additional device training. Nurses who receive extra training and provide support during the education process are good examples of potential super-users. They will help lead the education process and mentor those who need support, and will be a useful resource in the initial training, during refresher classes, and as support for new employees. One rule of thumb is to plan for one super-user for every 10 to 12 staff members who will need training.

Step 5: Define institution space and times for classes. Keep in mind that classes should be conducted within each shift during normal work hours. Asking people to stay after hours will create resentment and can compromise the success of your program. Each class should be announced in advance in order to give the nurse managers ample time to schedule class time for all nurses. And space is often at a premium in busy institutions, so be sure rooms are identified and reserved for your classes well ahead of time. Providing training sessions in the patient care area is most convenient for nurses and improves attendance.

Step 6: Promote the education process. To help everyone feel prepared and involved with the implementation of the new system, develop materials that describe how the education will proceed—who will attend what classes, when and where; what the classes will consist of; and why intelligent infusion technology is beneficial for patients, clinicians and the institution. Educational materials may consist of:
- Signs—posted throughout the hospital (including break rooms, nurses' stations).
- E-mail messages—reminders to individuals about upcoming classes, sign-up sheets to register for a training session, pump demonstrations with hands-on opportunity for the clinicians to practice with the new pumps, etc.
- Newsletters—regular communications that include interviews with people from other departments that describe their role in the implementation conversion; and interviews with health systems "officers" (CEO, CFO, CNO, CIO) and Director of Pharmacy to learn why it was important to switch

to the intelligent infusion devices. Promoting a culture of patient safety and specifically improving medication safety should be emphasized.

- Be creative—to generate interest and excitement, you may want to:
  - Create a graphic icon or theme for the conversion to intelligent infusion pumps; use it on posters, in newsletters, other communications.
  - Create a "diploma" or certificate that reflects successful training on the technology.
  - Other communication strategies!

Develop a Training Module

Before trying to tell others how to use the system, it is important for trainers to be sure the lessons presented are clear and concise. Guiding principles for the institution, described earlier (see Chapter 4) should be covered, including the medication and dose limitations (i.e., higher doses used in MICU vs. med/surg) available by critical care area, standardized processes by institution or each individual hospital of a health system, and changes in nurse processes that will occur with intelligent pump implementation. Training must include instruction on programming the device for a variety of drugs and doses, including scrolling the drug library for drug identification, steps for responding to hard and soft limit alerts, and infusion monitoring procedures/policies identifying that safety software use be mandatory so a compliance target can be identified (i.e., > 90%).

Be sure your training sessions are well planned, flexible, and mandatory. Your pump vendor may be able to provide educational materials to assist in your training needs. Also, develop easy-to-read support materials that cover the basics of pump usage as well as any new policies and procedures described in the training sessions. Nurses should be able to use these materials as reference while practicing on their own and even after the training sessions are over. If possible, post tutorials on the hospital website, so that users can continue to use the manuals after mandatory training is completed.

Provide Opportunities for Practice

It's one thing to listen to instructions and use the pumps in the classroom setting. It's another to do it in the clinical care areas on real patients. So that nurses can feel confident about their skills as they are learning, be sure to set aside a space where they can practice on pumps at their leisure and if possible have access to "super users" in case they have questions. Provide a specific training library that has been programmed into the pump. Typically, the training library will be used to demonstrate what types of alerts that users will commonly encounter. You will want alerts to fire during training sessions. But, alerts that are fired during training may also appear in your pump reports. Be sure to analyze initial reports for those doses entered and alerts fired that are "real," and did not occur during the training process. Your data will most certainly be skewed if alerts encountered during training are included in a performance improvement analysis.

Define Success

The facility should designate a supervisor who will "sign off" or "certify" that each nurse has been successfully trained in their ability to operate the new devices. Failure to achieve sign-off/certification should be followed by additional training and subsequent testing until satisfactory use is demonstrated. You may want to consider awarding a certificate of achievement when education is satisfactorily completed.

Prepare for "Go-Live"

The exact target day and time for going live will be determined by the project team. While education is proceeding, the rest of the intelligent infusion system is being set up and prepared for implementation. For example, policy and procedure must be developed, some processes standardized and others individualized for different care areas, drug libraries established, system uploads, and testing completed. The entire team may be involved with go-live, but on go-live day, nurses, materials management, biomedical personnel, and pharmacy may be especially affected.

It is important to map your go-live strategy in detail. This includes a deployment plan for conversion to the new pumps—will you go by clinical care area, by floor, or by campus? And where will you start? Some institutions begin with smaller units first and progress to specialized units (i.e., OR) last, to achieve success and to troubleshoot concerns during the process before moving on to larger, more complex clinical areas. Other institutions begin swapping out pumps in a few critical care areas and then halt the process for evaluation before proceeding to the rest of the institution. Because of the frequent transfer of patients between care areas and the movement of nurses between areas, some hospitals elect to do an entire hospital roll out of devices at one time after successful testing in a pilot test area.

Safety precautions are essential to assure that patient care continues uninterrupted. As each conventional pump is swapped out, accuracy of each infusion program on the intelligent pump must be confirmed before proceeding. This process for each pump should involve at least two persons, either two staff members or a staff member and a vendor representative assisting with the implementation process. Any questions or perceived issues should be communicated immediately to the super-user or project manager. The pharmacy department may need to obtain extra supplies for the pump "go-live," particularly if there are changes in infusion concentrations that will necessitate the "changing out" of infusion bags. Extra staffing may also be needed for the preparation of new infusion bags. Your hospital may have taken the opportunity presented by new pump implementation to standardize or change infusion concentrations. This may lead to confusion at the bedside. One tactic to deal with this problem is to include laminated cards that can attach to pump poles with basic instructions on pump programming, as well as standard infusion concentrations. Table 9-1 is an example of a card.

Because the "go-live" process affects the entire institution, it should be extensively communicated before the targeted conversion date. This helps create awareness and excitement, as well as prepare staff for the changes that will occur.

Go-Live Day

When the big day arrives, be sure all plans are in place.

Equipment. Pumps and appropriate tubing sets should be on hand. Special equipment needed in certain units (e.g., volumetric chambers sets in pediatrics) should also be readily available.

Teams. A go-live team made up of vendor representatives, a nurse educator, pharmacists, and materials management can lead the process. Multiple teams will be necessary for a hospital-wide roll-out.

Table 9-1. Common Infusion Concentrations and Rates, Abciximab (ReoPro)

Abciximab (ReoPro)
9 mg in 250 mL D5W (36 mcg/mL)
Initial bolus = 0.25 mg/kg (given over 5 minutes)
Continuous infusion = 0.125 mcg/kg/min if less than 80 kg

Weight kg/lb	Bolus Amount	Bolus Volume (over 5 minutes)	Infusion	Infusion Rate mL/hr
40/88	10 mg	5 mL	0.125 mcg/kg/min	8 mL/hr
45/99	11.2 mg	5.6 mL	0.125 mcg/kg/min	9 mL/hr
50/110	12.5 mg	6.2 mL	0.125 mcg/kg/min	10 mL/hr
55/121	13.8 mg	6.9 mL	0.125 mcg/kg/min	11 mL/hr
60/132	15 mg	7.5 mL	0.125 mcg/kg/min	12 mL/hr
65/143	16.2 mg	8.1 mL	0.125 mcg/kg/min	14 mL/hr
70/154	17.4 mg	8.7 mL	0.125 mcg/kg/min	15 mL/hr
75/165	18.8 mg	9.4 mL	0.125 mcg/kg/min	16 mL/hr
80/176	20 mg	10 mL	0.125 mcg/kg/min	17 mL/hr
85/187	21.2 mg	10.6 mL	10 mcg/min	17 mL/hr
90/198	22.4 mg	11.2 mL	10 mcg/min	17 mL/hr
95/209	23.8 mg	11.9 mL	10 mcg/min	17 mL/hr
100/220	25 mg	12.5 mL	10 mcg/min	17 mL/hr
105/231	26.2 mg	13.1 mL	10 mcg/min	17 mL/hr
110/242	27.4 mg	13.7 mL	10 mcg/min	17 mL/hr
115/253	28.8 mg	14.4 mL	10 mcg/min	17 mL/hr
120/264	30 mg	15 mL	10 mcg/min	17 mL/hr
125/275	31.2 mg	15.6 mL	10 mcg/min	17 mL/hr
130/286	32.4 mg	16.2 mL	10 mcg/min	17 mL/hr

Safety. These teams meet with a super-user in each unit to address safety issues for particular patients. You may want to prioritize swapping out based on pumps administering critical and/or multiple drips, and on infusion time remaining. Each unit needs to be aware of what time to expect the swap out to occur and they should be given about 15 minutes advanced notice before arrival. If possible a conversion per care area schedule should be in place and posted so each unit knows when to expect the implementation team to arrive.

Removal of old pumps and materials. To assure that all old pumps and tubing are removed, biomedical engineering (or other personnel), should keep track by recording serial numbers of the equipment as it is swapped out. Materials management (or other personnel) should replace tubing with new intelligent infusion pump tubing sets as or just before the pumps are converted. The unit manager should confirm that all pumps and old supplies have been removed from the unit and that new supplies are stocked and available for use.

Monitoring. Pharmacy should be ready to respond to questions or issues about drug libraries or dosing specifics as swapping out proceeds. Nurses, nurse educators, pharmacy, and other clinical personnel should be available to help manage specific patient issues and questions as they arise. Even early in the process after implementation, utilization reports (e.g., infusion summary or edit reports) can help identify issues that need to be addressed.

Are you ready? Be sure equipment, personnel, and safety measures are all in place

Evaluation and Assessment

Early after the implementation process, it is likely that the project team will collect baseline data that show current IV administration practices. These data help in the development and standardization of the drug libraries. But, very importantly the education team should work closely with pharmacy to assess efficacy once the intelligent infusion system is installed. Over time, you will be able to compare the effects of the intelligent infusion system with conventional pumps in preventing potential errors, identifying medication usage practices, safety software compliance, and reducing medication errors.

But in the near term, whether you implement a few critical care areas at a time, or the entire institution on a single day, it is important to closely monitor usage for a few days after implementation. Vendors will visit to assure that the system is working as planned, answer questions, and to assist in making any adjustments. The vendor can assist post implementation by assuring the staff are fully educated, they are using the pumps correctly, reports are being utilized to monitor compliance and the appropriateness of safety limits, and hand-off procedures and pump reprogramming is being done safely when patients are being moved from one level of care to another.

A thorough, well-thought-out education plan for go-live requires a strong commitment of time and resources by the institution and is essential to achieving the highest potential benefits of an intelligent safety software infusion system.

Educational classes should be mandatory for all nurses who will be using the new intelligent infusion pumps, refresher classes should be made available as needed, and super users must be available to support the clinicians while they develop a comfort level with using the new technology. Clinicians need to know and have continued reinforcement that upper management supports the use of the new technology to encourage a safe patient culture.

Be upbeat, positive, and excited. Change can be good, and this change will be good for the patients, the nurses, and the institution.

You will also receive support from intelligent infusion pump manufacturers. They will be able to offer suggestions and tools as you develop your education program. The vendor's experience in device implementation including user training, library build, driving compliance, and suggesting or providing tools to support the educational program is a valuable resource.

Conclusion

Many lessons can be learned before the implementation process that may improve prospects for high- and sustained compliance rates in use of the safety software. Education of the staff is crucial to making this transition a success. In this chapter you were given tips on how to develop the framework of an education plan in a step by step method, the creation of training modules and the post-implementation evaluation and assessment. Ongoing staff education and reinforcement of that education is vital in a multi-disciplinary environment.

PRACTICE TIPS

- Begin education of nurses at least 2 weeks prior to pump implementation.
- Supplement the formal learning process with additional tools and website materials.
- Conduct a "dry run" of the pump go-live on a particular patient care unit. Use what was learned from the "dry run" to improve your process and plan.
- Communication is critical. Once the nurses start the training, conduct weekly sessions to identify problems they have encountered.
- Be willing to make modifications in the drug library to address any issues identified during training.
- Be sure to "staff up" on go-live day, in order to ensure a smooth transition.

Suggested Reading

Adachi W, Lodolce AE. Use of failure mode and effects analysis in improving the safety of i.v. drug administration. *Am J Health-Syst Pharm*. 2005;62(9):917-920.

Cassano AT. IV medication safety software implementation in a multihospital health system. *Hosp Pharm*. 2006;41:151-156.

Siv-Lee, L, Morgan L. Implementation of wireless "intelligent" pump IV infusion technology in a not-for-profit academic setting. *Hosp Pharm*. 2007;42:832-840.

Wetterneck TB, Skibinski KA, Roberts TL, et al. Using failure mode and effects analysis to plan implementation of smart IV pump technology. *Am J Health-Syst Pharm*. 2006;63(16):1528-1538.

Special Drug Compounding

Craig E. Else, Carolyn Carlson, and
Virginia L. Ghafoor

Key Terms[1,2]

Bar code medication administration (BCMA)—technology that involves placing a unique identifier that is machine readable by an optical scanner on each medication.

Commercial product—sterile drug that has been evaluated by the Food and Drug Administration (FDA) for safety and efficacy.

Compounding—preparation, mixing, assembling, packaging, and labeling of a drug or device.

National drug code (NDC)—medication identity for commercial products which includes the drug company labeling, drug name, dose, and package size.

Introduction

Bar code medication administration (BCMA) has been shown to be effective in reducing medication errors before they reach the patient.[2] Parenteral (i.e., intravenous, IV) medication administration using smart pump technology requires bar code information on the product label for programming functions. Before medications are administered, BCMA matches the right medication with the right patient.

The extent of smart pump use is dependent on the availability of medications dispensed in packaging that fits the pump and recognition of the bar coded label by an optical scanner. Commercial parenteral products approved by the Food and Drug Administration (FDA) contain the National Drug Code number (i.e., NDC bar code) which may be suitable for some smart pumps. If the medication has an off-label use or concentration not commercially manufactured, pharmacy compounding and manual bar coding will be necessary.

There are many procedures associated with compounding medications for smart pumps. A decision will need to be made if the pharmacy will use commercially available parenteral solution or dry powder medications for compounding. If dry powders are used and/or extended dating is desired, quarantine procedures will need to be developed. Finally, after-hours procedures (if applicable) should be developed for pharmacy compounding.

Compounding

Parenteral medications administered via smart pump technology may be different from the normal stock vials in container size, volume, and concentration. Medication errors can occur with selection of the wrong drug or concentration during compounding of parenteral products. The errors that occur during preparation of the medication in the pharmacy will not be averted by bar code technology. Therefore, written procedures need to be established to reduce the risk of compounding errors in the pharmacy. A summit on preventing patient harm and death from intravenous medication errors by ASHP recommended priority safety practices. Table 10-1 provides a summary of recommendations pertinent to compounding medications for smart pumps.[3] This section will discuss processes for safe compounding, distribution, and storage of smart pump medications.

Concentration Choices

One of the decisions that will need to be made is whether to purchase premixed parenteral infusions and PCA syringes or bags from a manufacturer, or, compound parenteral products in the pharmacy. The Institute for Safe Medication Practices (ISMP) and the Joint Commission both recommend using manufactured products wherever available for safety and quality reasons.[2,4] While premixed products may be preferable, manufacturers often have limited products available for purchase

Table 10-1. Summary of Priority of IV Medication Safety Practices[3]

Formulary Management

- Implement standardized concentrations (dose, rate, units) based on local and national practices that are appropriate for most practice settings
- Use commercially available ready-to-administer medications if available
- Limit available concentrations of parenteral medication on the formulary
- Limit use of nonstandardized infusions to clinical indications in which benefits outweigh risks
- Implement hospital-wide standardized processes for high-alert medications

Storage and Dispensing

- Prohibit or impose tight security precautions on stocking concentration injectable projects and more than on concentration of an IV medication on patient care units
- Label IV products using standard format with prominent information needed by staff clearly identified
- Ensure competency of pharmacists and technicians who prepare IV medication
- Use best practices for preparation of IV products in addition to practices for assuring stability and sterility in USP chapter 797[1]
- Use machine-readable codes to verify accuracy of medication dispensing and filling of automated dispensing cabinets (ADCs)

with new technology due to FDA approval limits for the device. Many of the new smart pumps are approved for administration of commercially available products. An alternative to purchasing commercial products is to either compound them internally or outsource compounding to an admixture pharmacy. Advantages of internally compounding include flexibility of medications and concentrations, low cost, and direct control and oversight of the compounding process. Reasons for outsourcing compounding include standardization, improved quality control, decreased labor and extended product dating.

Non-standard drug concentrations will need to be compounded in the pharmacy for certain patient populations. These concentrations should be identified, standardized, and processes developed to safely and efficiently compound and dispense them.[1,3] As an example, hydromorphone 10 mg/mL and morphine 25 mg/mL are commercially available in vials but not PCA products. Concentrated opioids should be reserved high-dose cancer or chronic pain patients. Justification for compounding highly concentrated parenteral opioids is twofold because:

- Use of standard PCA opioid concentrations to deliver high opioid doses may exceed the pump's capacity for flow rate.
- Using large volume bags or frequently changing PCA syringes is not optimal patient care.

Since high concentrations will be rarely used, rigorous compounding processes should be developed including specialized storage, unique labeling, and double checks during preparation.[1,5,6] Figure 10-1 is an example high risk compounding procedure.

Product:

Hydromorphone 1 mg/mL in 30-mL vial for Hospira LifeCare PCA Pump

Supplies:

- Ordered medication in sufficient quantity
- Diluent in sufficient quantity, if required
- Appropriate barcode label (located with medication in CII safe)
- 60-mL syringe, and needle; syringe and needle for diluent if required
- Syringe-to-syringe adaptor
- 30-mL sterile empty vial and injector
- Sterile yellow vial cap
- Tamper evident-tape
- Patient name label

Procedure:

Following standard operating procedures for compounded sterile preparations including cleaning, garb, and aseptic technique, gather the supplies in the IV hood and prepare to compound.

1. Remove the sterile empty vial from its packaging. Twist the injector clockwise to engage the needle. Depress the injector to remove any air from the end of the vial.
2. Using the 60-mL syringe and needle, withdraw the appropriate volume of the ordered medication from the manufacturer vials/ampules. Remove the needle.
3. If dilution is needed, withdraw the appropriate amount of diluent from the manufacturer container in a separate syringe. Then add the diluent to the
4. medication in the 60-mL syringe, draw back on the plunger to create a 5-mL air bubble, cap with rubber cap and mix thoroughly. Remove the cap and the air bubble.
5. Attach the syringe-to-syringe connector to the 60-mL syringe containing the medication.
6. Remove the yellow cap from the luer-lock end of the injector. Connect the other end of the syringe-to-syringe connector to the luer-lock on the injector.
7. Keeping the assembly in a vertical orientation with the vial on the bottom, depress the syringe plunger and fill the vial with 30 mL of the ordered medication. A small air bubble may be present in the vial, and does NOT have to be removed.
8. Disconnect the syringe and adaptor from the injector. Unscrew the injector from the blue rubber stopper, and discard in sharps bin. Place a sterile yellow cap on the vial.
9. Write the appropriate lot number and 48-hour expiration date on the barcode label, and initial patient label
10. Give source vial(s), pulled back syringe(s) showing amount of medication and diluent used, finished PCA vial and labels to pharmacist for checking.
11. Pharmacist checks source vial(s) and volume of medication added to PCA vial, and if correct initials the patient name label.
12. Affix tamper-evident tape to secure cap to PCA vial on two sides. It is important to do this before adding other labels to the vial, so that information is not covered by the tamper tape. Affix barcode and patient name labels to vial.

Figure 10-1. Example of high concentration PCA procedure.

Standardization

The most successful strategy you can pursue regarding pump implementation is to standardize concentrations as much as possible. Standardization improves patient safety, decreases costs and improves operational efficiencies.[3,5] Patient safety is improved through decreased risk of inadvertent preparation, dispens-

ing or administration of an incorrect concentration. The fewer concentrations available, the chance is lower an error can occur.[4]

To avoid mis-programming the pump, the pharmacy label should read exactly as the medication name in the pump programming. For example, if you have set up a medication name in the pump as "dopamine—high dose," then the pharmacy label should exactly match that naming convention. This precaution will help to avoid choosing the wrong drug and concentration in the pump library.

Product Quality and Sterility

Compounding of parenteral preparations should follow requirements as outlined in USP's Chapter 797.[1,6] Many of the products used will be low or medium risk products per USP797 definitions.[1] Some facilities may decide to batch compound commonly used products. If extended dating is needed, processes for quality testing and quarantine should be developed. Similarly, high risk compounded products such as high concentration infusions prepared from dry powders should have similar policies and procedures developed to ensure quality and safety.[1]

Label Generation

Equipment will need to be obtained to print labels with both barcodes and text. An ideal label printer will be easy to operate and format and will produce durable labels that can be clearly and consistently read by the barcode reader. It is very important to ensure that labels are produced that are the correct format and size to be read by the barcode reader. Select a printer that has user-friendly software for formatting barcode and text size, as well as position on the label. The labels should be resistant to damage from moisture and scratches from handling, packaging or use with the pump.

Bar codes may be produced at the time of dispensing or compounding, or may be pre-printed. If labels are needed at multiple sites within the same health care system, it may be most cost-effective to pre-print labels at a central location for distribution to the various sites. If labels are pre-printed, a process should be developed to ensure that the correct label is selected; this can include storing each type of label with its respective drug and building in pharmacist double-checks of barcode selection.

Generally, compounding labels should include pharmacy name, drug name and concentration with corresponding barcode, lot or control number and the proper expiration date.[1] Be sure that all labels fulfill the requirements of current state and federal laws. Information about the drug name and concentration on the label should exactly match the entry in the drug library so that there is no confusion when programming the pump. For example, if hydromorphone 10 mg/mL is called "Hydromorphone Non-Std Conc" in the drug library, the barcoded label should also read "Hydromorphone Non-Std Conc." Patient-specific information may be printed on the barcode label as well, although it may be easier to print this information on a separate label, especially if the compounding labels are being pre-printed.

Use of auxiliary labels, especially for non-standard or high concentration drugs, should be consistent; it should be pre-determined which drugs or concentrations require auxiliary labels. Auxiliary labels of standardized text, color and size should be used so that they can easily be recognized by staff administering the medications.

Finally, it is important to follow any pump-specific guidelines for placement of the barcode label. This is necessary for both safety and efficiency.[2] It may be helpful to provide an example or diagram of a final product with correct barcode label placement to staff who will be labeling or checking the products.

Storage

Storage may be needed in several different areas of the facility. Compounding supplies, including drug vials, barcodes and/or printers, compounding instructions and checklists and any special equipment needed for the particular pump, will likely need to be stored in or near the central pharmacy. Additional space may be needed in the IV room, in refrigerators or in secure narcotics storage. Supplies should be readily available in case of "stat" orders.

Additionally, the final products will need to be stored and secured. Any narcotic vaults or automatic dispensing cabinets that are to be used will need adequate space set aside to fit the products in their final compounded forms. It may be helpful to determine past usage of the products to be dispensed in the facility to estimate the volume that will need to be stored. Special product packaging (wraps, bags, caps, tamper-resistant devices, attached tubing or plungers, etc.) should be taken into consideration when determining the space needed.

Stat/After-Hours Orders

Policies should be developed concerning when and how quickly products are expected to be dispensed and/or compounded. Some things to take into consideration include: staffing, equipment availability, time needed to compound and check products properly, and current expectations for providing "stat" medications. If pharmacy services are limited during certain hours of the day, policies should be developed to handle orders that are written at these times; this may need to include temporary substitution of another pre-made product.

Training

Training will need to be provided to technicians, pharmacists and any other personnel that will be a part of the process of compounding, labeling or dispensing these products.[1,6] Compounding demonstrations, review of standardized compounding instructions and examples of properly compounded and labeled products may be included in the training of technicians and pharmacists. Refer

Pharmacist Double-Checklist		
Date:		
Patient Name:		
Medical Record Number:		
Drug:	**Concentration:**	
Item to Check:	**RPh 1**	**RPh 2**
Correct drug vial displayed		
Correct barcode selected and properly placed		
Correct diluent displayed		
Syringes pulled back to correct volume added		
Patient label affixed properly		
Auxiliary label affixed for non-standard concentrations		
Correct expiration on label		
Injector removed; cap secured with tamper-evident tape		
Time of Check:		

Figure 10-2. Non-standard PCA preparation checklist.

to Figure 10-1 for an example compounding procedure. In addition, pharmacists should be trained to properly check (and/or double-check) products and complete any required documentation.[1,5] Figure 10-2 is an example of documentation.

Conclusion

Compounding parenteral products for smart pump administration is necessary if the medication and /or concentration is not commercially available in a container size suitable for the device. There are many processes associated with compounding medications for smart pumps including product preparation, manual bar coding of the label, and storage in automated dispensing cabinets. Written procedures need to be established to reduce the risk of compounding errors in the pharmacy. Pharmacy staff need to be trained on the compounding procedures, labeling and dispensing of these products. Clinical management will need to establish policy expectations for providing "stat" medications that require custom compounding.

PRACTICE TIPS

- Analyze commercially available products to avoid excessive product compounding.
- Understand the bar-coding capabilities of the pump you have chosen.
- Standardize dosages and concentrations as much as possible.
- Understand USP 797 product quality and storage requirements.
- If you intend to compound and bar-code label medications, a special printer will likely need to be purchased.
- Develop checklists for preparation that include double-check requirements and signature requirements.
- Develop procedures for after-hours compounding.

References

1. The Pharmacopeia of the United States of America, 32nd revision and the National Formulary, 27th ed. May 1, 2009.

2. Cochran GL, Jones KJ, Brockman J, Skinner A, Hicks RW. Errors prevented by and associated with bar-code medication administration systems. *Jt Comm J Qual Patient Saf.* 2007;33(5):293-301.

3. Proceedings of a summit on preventing patient harm and death from IV medication errors. *Am J Health-Syst Pharm.* 2008;65:2367-2379.

4. Misprogramming PCA Concentration Leads to Dosing Errors. Institute for Safe Medication Practices Newsletter. August 28, 2008. Available at: http://www.ismp.org/newsletters.

5. Oishi R. Current status of preparation and distribution of medicines. *Am J Health-Syst Pharm.* 2009; 66(1):Suppl S35-S42.

6. Kastango ES. Blueprint for implementing USP chapter 797 for compounding sterile preparations. *Am J Health-Syst Pharm.* 2005;62:1272-1288.

Updating the Drug Library and Implementing System Changes

Susan M. Kleppin

Key Terms

Smart infusion pumps—a new generation of infusion pumps that incorporates dose limiting software into the pump hardware; this software is designed to prevent infusion-related programming errors. The Joint Commission, in the 2006 National Patient Safety Goals, defined a smart pump as a "parenteral infusion pump equipped with IV medication error-prevention software that alerts operators or interrupts the infusion process when a pump setting is programmed outside of pre-configured limits. Smart pumps are designed to recognize prescription errors, dose misinterpretations, and keypad programming errors."

Drug library—a comprehensive list of medications and fluids that are to be delivered using the infusion pump. This library includes any dose, volume, or rate limitations that are programmed into the software.

Drug dataset—used interchangeably with drug library (see above).

Introduction

As discussed earlier in this book, implementation of intelligent infusion device technology requires the collaboration and communication of a multidisciplinary team. Once the technology is implemented, the work is not done. Changes after implementation such as updates to the drug library in the infusion device or software updates that will affect practice and infusion device utilization require the oversight of a dedicated group or team.

Continuing the Multidisciplinary Team Approach

After intelligent infusion device technology has been implemented, it is wise to identify a group of individuals from a variety of disciplines that will continue to serve in an advisory role should changes to drug libraries, pump policies or procedures, or related technology adoption be pursued in the future. Ideally, the membership of the advisory group will be similar to that used as the infusion device technology was implemented. Suggested members include representatives from nursing, pharmacy, biomedical engineering, central services (or department responsible for distribution and cleaning of infusion devices), plant engineering and information systems. In addition, ad hoc members to the advisory group may be necessary if the changes planned will affect other practitioners. For example, the adoption of modular patient controlled analgesia technology that is integrated with the infusion device might require that anesthesiologists and pain care specialists serve as ad hoc members of the advisory group. The role of each of these departments is dependent upon the upgrade that is planned; in some cases, each department may not have a role in the planned upgrade. Ideally, this group should be led by a single individual who will assume responsibility for coordination of meetings and communication between the disciplines. If your hospital has a nursing-led venous access team, an individual from this group may be a good choice as project lead. Alternatively, the group could be led by a pair of individuals; for example, a nursing representative and a pharmacy representative could work together to lead an upgrade project. It is recommended that the advisory group's members be identified and a roster of the members and their contact information be maintained and distributed to all members. Frequent updates may be necessary, as individual's roles in the organization change. This will facilitate easy communication between all departments should a project be planned by any department that might affect infusion device utilization.

Each department represented in the advisory group has a distinct role in any upgrade being planned. The nursing representation should include both clinicians who work with the infusion devices on a daily basis as well as nursing education specialists, if such a position exists at your hospital, to facilitate education of the front-line nursing staff. Pharmacy representation should include the individual who is responsible for the maintenance of the drug library. Representation from the biomedical engineering department is suggested as these individuals are responsible for the repair and maintenance of the infusion devices. The hospital department responsible for distribution of the devices should be included in the advisory group as employees in that department may need to assist in any upgrade planned and are also likely responsible for any rental infusion devices that are utilized by the hospital. The hospital department responsible for cleaning of the infusion devices should be included in the advisory group or as an ad hoc member as employees will be responsible for cleaning of any new infusion equipment and would also be involved in the cleaning of equipment that has been upgraded or serviced prior to recirculation for patient care. Lastly, the information technology services department has a role in the advisory group should radio frequency technology be used for pump communication or if integration with bar code technology or computerized physician order entry be planned.

When updates to the pump technology are planned, the advisory group can be called into action to manage the process. It is recommended that the hospital have procedures developed and in place to outline the process by which changes will be managed. The project lead should have the responsibility for meeting coordination, agenda development, project timeline development, and assignment of responsibilities. Checklist development can be helpful to ensure that all necessary tasks have been completed prior to implementation of the planned change.

Drug Library Updates

When modifications are made to the drug dataset, consideration should be given to enlisting the help of the advisory group as well as any ad hoc members that are necessary. A method should be in place to compile suggestions for drug dataset modifications. These suggestions could be submitted by any clinician in the facility and might be necessary because of medication formulary changes (additions or deletions), changes in practice or in the type of patients being cared for, a review of the continuous quality improvement data from the pumps, or the addition of new equipment. It is recommended that the suggestions for modifications be forwarded to one individual who will take responsibility for tracking suggestions and ensuring that they are considered for appropriateness. Ideally, this individual should be a nurse or a pharmacist who has both clinical expertise as well as knowledge of pump operation.

Hospital policy and procedure should be established as to how dataset modifications are to be approved. A variety of approaches might be used. Ideally, the approval process should include a check of accuracy and appropriateness for the modification being programmed. Review by clinicians is essential and might include nurses, pharmacists, and physicians. One approach to the approval process would be to have the hospital's Pharmacy and Therapeutics Committee be responsible for review of proposed changes to the dataset. A subcommittee of the Pharmacy and Therapeutics Committee could also be charged with this responsibility; for example, a hospital's medication safety committee could be responsible. Other options for review and approval of proposed dataset modifications would be to enlist the assistance of a nursing/pharmacy committee, a nursing practice committee, or another hospital committee. Regardless of the approach utilized, it is essential that the proposed changes undergo a multidisciplinary review.

When drug library modifications are made, the hospital will also need to consider whether existing order sets need modification as well. If the hospital utilizes an electronic medical record that includes flowsheets for IV infusions, consideration will need to be given to whether or not the flowsheets need revision. If the hospital utilizes tall-man lettering for look-alike/sound-alike medication names, this should also be incorporated into any drug library modifications and the labels of IV admixtures should be similar to the pump display to further prevent programming errors.

Hospital procedure or policy can dictate how often drug dataset changes are made. The frequency with which changes are made will be dependent on several factors.

- First, a change in practice or a formulary change may require a more immediate response.
- Second, the urgency of the request is considered. If changes are needed to avoid harm to patients due to an FDA decision or warning, these of course should be handled immediately.
- Third, frequency may be influenced by the method with which the dataset is transferred to the pump software.

If your hospital uses radio-frequency technology to transfer the dataset to the pump software, it is much easier and faster to make more frequent changes to the dataset. If radio-frequency technology is not in use, the transfer of the dataset to the pump software is much more labor-intensive and time consuming, as pumps must be physically returned, connected to a computer and the new dataset downloaded onto the pump.

When dataset modifications are ready to be downloaded to the pump hardware, there are several things that the advisory group should consider. How will the changes being made to the dataset be communicated to end-users? This communication/education may be essential for some changes (i.e., addition of new drugs or profiles) and may not be as necessary for others (i.e., modification of infusion rates). Collaboration between the nursing and pharmacy departments will be essential to determine if education or communication is necessary and how it might be best accomplished.

Radio Frequency Transfer

The method of transfer of the dataset to the pump hardware will dictate when and how the transfer will occur. If radio frequency technology is being used to communicate with the pumps, scheduling the dataset transfer will be easy. A date and time can be chosen so that monitoring of the dataset transfer via the server can be accomplished easily. The date and time chosen should be communicated to the advisory group so that all disciplines involved are aware of the plan. It is recommended that a member of the advisory group be responsible for electronically monitoring the dataset transfer to ensure that no problems are encountered and to monitor the progress of the transfer. Any pumps being stored or utilized outside of radio frequency range will either need to be brought back into range to allow for the dataset transfer or arrangements made to transfer the dataset manually.

Manual Transfer

If radio frequency technology is not being used, a more elaborate plan will need to be developed for the circulation of pump equipment from patient care areas to a central location to allow for this manual download process. It is necessary to ensure that all pumps have the most current dataset on them. This may necessitate the "swapping out" of equipment that is currently in use on patients. This manual process will require extensive coordination with nursing, biomedical engineering, and central services (or department responsible for distribution and cleaning of infusion devices). Pumps removed from patient care areas for the dataset transfer will likely need to be cleaned before the process can begin for infection control purposes. Hospital policy may dictate that the pumps are cleaned again after the transfer prior to being returned to use. This also may be a good opportunity to do preventive maintenance on the pumps. Depending on how much pump equipment a hospital has, this manual dataset transfer could take several days to several weeks. A method to track which devices have the new dataset will need to be utilized to ensure that all infusion devices have been updated.

Regardless of which method is used for the dataset transfer, an electronic copy of the new dataset should be forwarded to the biomedical engineering department. This copy of the dataset will need to be utilized should the hospital need to lease additional pump equipment for some reason or after a device is serviced if a dataset needs to be uploaded.

Software Upgrade

Should the decision be made to upgrade the software version on the intelligent infusion devices, the hospital will have to develop a plan for circulation of pump equipment from patient care areas to a central location for the upgrade. Typically, a software upgrade in the intelligent infusion devices cannot be accomplished via radio frequency; it requires a manual upload of the updated software version to the pump and any auxiliary modules. Just as with the manual dataset transfer, the "swapping out" of equipment that is currently in use on patients may be necessary. This manual process will require extensive coordination with nursing, biomedical engineering, and central services (or department responsible for distribution and cleaning of infusion devices) and could take several days to several weeks. A method to track which devices have the new software will need to be utilized to ensure that all infusion devices have been updated.

A software version upgrade also requires more extensive end-user education as the software likely offers enhancements and changes in functionality of the pump. A thorough education plan will need to be developed for the nursing staff and physicians who routinely use the pumps. Pharmacists who work in patient care areas will also need to be made aware of the changes and any impact it might have on them.

New Technology Adoption

The advisory group will likely also need to be involved with the purchase and implementation of any new intelligent infusion pump technology (i.e., syringe module addition) or with the integration of the infusion pump technology with other patient care technology, such as bar code administration or computerized physician order entry technology (CPOE). These processes will require extensive collaboration and cooperation between multiple departments in the hospital. These types of implementations will also require much more education for end-users and an extensive education plan will need to be developed. Consideration needs to be given to how long before the implementation of the new technology the training sessions should be completed, to the training methods that will be employed, and a decision made as to whether competency assessment will be necessary prior to implementation.

Supplier/Manufacturer Support

Fortunately, the manufacturers of intelligent infusion device technology have well developed implementation processes for new and existing customers and guide hospital personnel through device upgrade or new technology implementation. As a rule, a project manager employed by the manufacturer of the infusion device will be assigned to work with a project manager and team from the hospital to work on the implementation plan. The manufacturer will likely contribute administrative support and assistance with organizing/guiding the team that will be completing the work. In addition, the manufacturers of the intelligent infusion devices are usually willing to share data and experiences from other hospitals, which can be very helpful. Vendors may also supply training for personnel who are responsible for dataset management and pump repair and maintenance. Ongoing support programs are usually available and part of the original purchase agreements and can be extremely helpful as changes are made in equipment utilization or as personnel changes occur.

Conclusion

A multidisciplinary team approach is necessary to address any modifications to the drug dataset and/or implementation of new pump technology or integration with other error reduction technologies. A great deal of attention to detail is required to manage such projects to ensure that the changes are carried out methodically and accurately to prevent any inadvertent errors.

PRACTICE TIPS

- Plan ahead for pump updates: identify a lead group to manage the pump and library upgrades.
- Identify approval process for pump library changes.
- Identify the impact of pump library changes on the electronic medical record, the eMAR, the flowsheets, and any order sets.
- Pump tracking is essential during a pump library update; you will need to be able to track which pumps have the new library or software on them, and which have the old version.
- Identify a team of pharmacists and nurses to conduct the pump "swap." This may include the preparation of new infusion bags.
- Practicing a "dry run" of library or software updates ahead of time will identify any issues and challenges in the updates.

Suggested Reading

Sanborn M, Cohen T. Get smart: effective use of smart pump technology. *Hosp Pharm.* 2009;44;348-353.

Wetterneck TB, Skibinski KA, Roberts TL, et al. Using failure mode and effects analysis to plan implementation of smart i.v. pump technology. *Am J Health-Syst Pharm.* 2006;63:1528-1538.

Monitoring Quality and Pump Utilization

Burnis D. Breland

Key Terms

Clinical care area (also called CCA or drug library subset)—an area of the health system representing a certain group of patients who have similar patient care needs. For purposes of the infusion pump, a clinical care area is part of the pump programming that allows medications needed in the particular area to be separated into one particular list for one particular area. One example of a clinical care area is an "intensive care unit."

DERS or safety software—a term used to describe software built into intelligent infusion devices that is designed to catch dosing or administration errors. In this case, it represents the programming of minimum and maximum dose limits in an infusion pump, and the alerts presented to the clinician when programmed doses are exceeded.

"Hard" dose limit—a dose limit programmed into a pump; the pump cannot be programmed outside a "hard" limit. The user must use a dose within the hard limits.

Overrides—the action of continuing to program the pump at the bedside with entered doses, concentrations, or rates despite receiving high or low dose alerts.

Pump edits—the action of modifying pump programming at the bedside in response to a high or low dose alert.

"Soft" dose limit—a dose limit programmed into a pump; the pump will alert the user that the dose is unusual, however, the user can still proceed with programming this dose.

Introduction

One of the most valuable features of an intelligent infusion system is the report data that comes out of the safety software. Standard reports provide a wealth of information about how pumps are used, which drugs are prescribed most often, where compliance is low (or high), what drug doses are routinely overridden, and what types of infusion edits are occurring and how frequently. If more specific information is required then you may need to work with your vendor to obtain additional reports. With these data, managers will have a clear picture of IV infusion administration practices in their institution, and will be able to identify policies or procedures that may need to be reassessed and/or improved. And the reports are essential in developing and monitoring CQI (continuous quality improvement) initiatives such as standardizing medication administration practices with appropriate dose and rates of infusion.

So where do you start?

Assign a Team

First, be sure that a task force or team is identified to discuss and decide the kinds of information needed, how the reports can meet these needs, and how and by whom data collection and analysis will be managed. This team should include pharmacists and nurses, but might also include risk management, quality management, biomedical, or other personnel (e.g., IS representative).

Initiate Discussions Early

It may seem counterintuitive to talk about reports—which are, after all, an endpoint in the IV administration process—before the system has even been installed. But the earlier you think about what kinds of information your institution wants to collect on an *ongoing basis* the more time and cost-effective your system will prove to be. Recognizing what reports will be available, understanding what the data from the reports are conveying, being able to accurately interpret the reports and being prepared to act on the data is all very important.

- Become familiar with standard reports. These include:
  - *Infusion summary report*—provides a summary of infusion activity (compliance with use of safety software, overrides, and edits); can be run by infuser type (i.e., general infusion or PCA), clinical care area (CCA), or a select time period.
  - *Edit variance report*—provides a line-item detail of every infusion program in which a clinician edited the program in response to an alert; can be run by CCA, medication, selected CCAs or medications, or all CCAs or medications.
  - *Override variance details report*—provides a line-item detail of every infusion program where the user received an alert and chose to continue with the

initially entered value; can be run by CCA, medication, selected CCAs or medications, or all CCAs and medications.

- *Medications infused by CCA report*—provides detailed information on clinician responses to alerts for individual medications; can be run by CCA, medication, or service line.
- *Infusion status report*—provides pharmacists and nurse managers with real-time information to monitor infusions and to follow up on those running outside of the facility defined limits or those running with no safety limits; can be grouped by CCA or medication.
- *Asset tracker report*—provides information that helps efficiently manage the entire inventory of infusers, identifies the version of the library installed, and identifies the device's last location while running.

> **Note:** The report names listed here are specific to one vendor. Check with your pump vendor to identify which reports are the same as, or similar to the ones listed above.

- From these reports you will be able to learn, among other things:
  - Which medications are used most often in a specific care area; what medications might be missing from the drug library, or whether the drug library needs to be modified.
  - Frequency of soft-limit overrides.
  - Incidence of "near misses"—edits that prevented a potential medication error.
  - Near real-time status of a given infusion.
  - Pump location (last access point the device communicated with).
  - Library update status of individual pumps.
  - Comparison of infusion practices across facilities within an institution.
  - Compliance with the use of safety software.
  - Hard limit attempts.

Identify a Reports Manager

This person should be part of the task force team. This is one job that will continue long after implementation has been completed. Therefore, the candidate's job requirements should be revised to accommodate the new responsibilities, including supervision of data collection for the reports, reports analysis, and distribution of the findings to appropriate personnel (e.g., pharmacy leaders, nursing, website) on a regular basis. Individual patient care area managers should be made aware in a timely manner of infusion practices in order to improve safe and effective medication practices.

The team should have a discussion regarding who will have access to the reports. If only one person has access, the information is not necessarily disseminated in a timely fashion. Some institutions elect to post data on the facility website; the data is transparent for all to view. Ideally, greater transparency will lead to better understanding and results. Nurse managers and nursing leadership should have open access to reports for their staff and patient care units. Performance Improvement staff may also want to access the reports for institution performance measurement.

- *Identify the reports framework.* Every institution has different requirements, but the reporting software must be flexible enough to meet a wide range of needs. That is why it is important to think through carefully how the reports will be used, so that the information provided can help optimize safety and quality of care in your institution. These decisions will take time and may change as use of the intelligent infusion system evolves. Among issues the team should consider are:
    - Which reports do you want to use? Are the standard reports adequate? Or is more specific information required on the facilities medication use process? If so, you may be able to work with your vendor to obtain more specialized reports.
    - How frequently should reports be generated? This depends on the type of reports you select and what you want to achieve.

        Within 30 days of implementation, it is recommended that you generate reports to determine safety software compliance and to detect any issues with the drug library (e.g., inappropriate dosing limits, and missing drugs). After that, you can generate reports weekly, bi-weekly, monthly, or on whatever schedule provides the information you want to monitor IV infusion administration in your institution. Consider that you will probably want to compare some data over time—for example, compliance between clinical care areas or at the facility level from one quarter to the next, or frequency of overrides between clinical care areas from one month to the next.
- *Decide how data will be shared with staff.* First of all, keep in mind that the reports are not intended to be "gotcha" tools. Staff should not be made to feel that someone is waiting to catch them making a mistake. The ideal environment is one that is not punitive in nature to encourage clinicians to report events in the hopes the facility can learn from its mistakes. Help them understand that the reports are intended to support quality care and to benefit the patient, the caregiver, and the institution. That is why the data are collected and analyzed—so current practices can be improved upon. How the data are shared will go a long way to making intelligent infusion devices a success in your institution.

- Regularly scheduled meetings. Many institutions share results during regular staff meetings—they demonstrate and discuss where improvement has been made, how a goal has been reached, and what other initiatives need to be implemented.
- Posting. Institutions should post the results regularly as a kind of "cheer-leading" tool to identify goals achieved (e.g., improved compliance). Posting in a prominent place allows staff to see the results at their own convenience, and promotes awareness of how these intelligent infusion devices impact quality of care every day.
- Private sessions. If compliance or another issue is of particular concern for certain personnel, a private meeting to discuss report results may be advisable. Remember, the focus of the reports is to make improvements, not to assign blame.

- *Use reports on an ongoing basis.* Reports can help the clinicians see how the technology has assisted in reducing medication errors, improve quality of care, potentially lower costs, and support asset management and CQI initiatives. In addition, reports can also be a great confidence-builder and morale-enhancer for your staff when they see in black and white that goals were achieved, issues were solved and harm to the patient was prevented.

It may take some weeks or months to determine exactly how frequently you want to generate reports and how often you share the results. But if you establish and publicize reports on a regular basis, you can create anticipation and excitement among the staff, who will look forward to seeing how they've contributed to improved IV infusion administration in their institution.

Following are sample standard reports and analyses that give you an idea of how the data can be interpreted (see Figure 12-1) Note the details that are available, and the ease in data compilation. For more examples, and to discuss specific needs of your institution, contact your vendor.

Conclusion

Reports generated from the intelligent infusion software are invaluable tools for managing, monitoring, and improving the therapeutics and safety of IV infusion administration. Select and manage the reports structure as carefully as you build your drug libraries. The payoffs will continue for years to come.

Infusion Summary

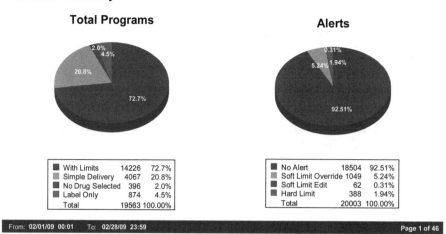

| | | | | Edit Variance Detail | | | |
	Alert Date/Time	**Limit**	**Limit Violated**	**Initial Dose**	**Final Dose**	**Variance**
CCA: 7 MAIN						
Heparin 25000 units/250 mL	09/05/2007 05:52:24	50 units/hr	• lower soft	12	1200	-76.00%
CCA: 8 MAIN						
Enalaprilat (Vasotec)	07/30/2007 11:39:51	50 mL/hr	• UPPER SOFT	100	50	100.00%
Heparin 25000 units/250 mL	07/31/2007 11:50:34	50 units/hr	• lower soft	12.5	12.5	-75.00%
Heparin 25000 units/250 mL	08/02/2007 19:08:36	50 units/hr	• lower soft	12.5	1250	-75.00%
CCA: 8ICU						
Nicardipine 25 mg/250 mL	08/18/2007 04:10:02	9 mg/hr	• UPPER SOFT	11	1	22.22%
CCA: LD						
Oxytocin 500 mL	07/26/2007 06:54:18	20 mL/hr	• UPPER SOFT	22	2	10.00%
Oxytocin 500 mL	09/19/2007 12:47:16	20 mL/hr	• UPPER SOFT	56	6	180.00%
CCA: 7ICU						
Norepinephrine 8 mg/250 mL	12/13/2007 17:59:35	20 mcg/min	• UPPER SOFT	100	10	400.00%

Figure 12-1. Edit variance detail report.

PRACTICE TIPS

- **Who is on the team?** Pharmacists, nurses, risk management, quality, biomedical, and other personnel (i.e., IT representative).
- **When to start?** Before system implementation.
- **The reports manager's job.** Continues long after system implementation.
- **The reports framework.** Decide on what reports to use, how often to generate them, and how to the share results.
- **The role of reports in managing intelligent infusion.** Reports should be used continuously and shared with the end users of the devices.

Case Studies

Case Study #1

Two months after large volume pumps have been implemented, a report is generated that shows that the intensive care unit routinely overrides the dexmedetomidine soft limit. Upon further investigation, managers discover that the medical staff is using the drug at high doses to reduce narcotic utilization. Doses of dexmedetomidine used are substantiated by literature; the alerts are merely causing a nuisance to the nursing staff and providing no benefit to patient care. The end result is to raise the soft limit to a higher level to avoid nuisance alerts. This situation may occur quite frequently during the initial phase of implementation.

Case Study #2

An institution implements new large volume pumps. A quarterly report is generated that shows how many dose "edits" occurred during the quarter. The report identifies doses that were modified as a result of pump alerts. The institution can also see the magnitude of the potential dosing error, and assign a severity of the adverse event that might have occurred. For more severe events, a dollar value cost avoidance (consistent with literature values) can be calculated. The institution uses this figure in the original return on investment (ROI) analysis to show that the pumps are "paying for themselves." This information should be communicated to institution senior leadership and the institution board of directors as an example of a successful technology implementation. Celebrating the "good catches" with staff also reinforces the value of the smart pump technology and the value of using the safety software.

Case Study #3

A nurse manager is concerned about whether or not the staff on the unit is using the safety software, and how many limits are overridden. The manager generates a real-time report at the start of each shift. The manager conducts "pump rounds" to identify what issues are causing nurses to work outside of the safety limits. In this manner, the nuisance alerts can be identified and eliminated, education regarding the pump safety features can occur on the spot, and the expectation of compliance with safety software can be imparted.

Case Study #4

A nurse manager discovers from shift-specific reports that the night shift is working outside of the drug library ("no drug selected" or "other drug") more frequently than the other shifts. The manager holds meetings with the staff to discover what barriers exist to the staff using the safety software. Some of the staff members were on vacation during the training period and are confused with the operation of the pump. Training is completed and staff become compliant with use of the safety software. One staff member, however, complains that he doesn't want to do the extra steps to program the pump and refuses to comply. The manager may need to go into a performance management process with this individual.

Case Study #5

Shortly after implementation, managers are shocked to discover a very high rate of hard limits that are reached in pump programming. Upon further investigation, they discover that the hard limits reached are in the "training" library or the "demonstration" library. Clearly, the training library will serve to show users how the alerts work, and therefore abnormally high doses will routinely be entered. The data from the training library should intentionally be eliminated from any performance improvement reports.

Suggested Reading

Breland D. Continuous quality improvement using intelligent infusion pump data analysis. *Am J Health-Syst Pharm.* 2010;67:1446-1455.

Pedersen CA, Gumpper KF. ASHP national survey on informatics: assessment of the adoption and use of pharmacy informatics in U.S. hospitals—2007. *Am J Health-Syst Pharm.* 2008;65(23):2244-2264.

ISMP's list of high-alert medications. Available at: http://www.ismp.org/Tools/highalertmedications.pdf . Accessed April 15, 2009.

Wilson K, Sullivan M. Preventing medication errors with smart infusion technology. *Am J Health-Syst Pharm.* 2004;61:177-183.

Danello SH, Maddox RR, Schaack GJ. Intravenous infusion safety technology: return on investment. *Hosp Pharm.* 2009;44:680.

Checklists for Go-Live and Updates

Pamela K. Phelps, Janell M. Schultz,
Carol S. Manchester, and Gregg F. Herrmann

Key Terms

Biomedical services—department within the health system concerned with storing and maintaining biomedical equipment and technology.

DL—drug library.

Drug library push—the act of updating pumps using wireless technology. The new drug library is "pushed" from the software housing the library out to the individual pumps.

EMR—electronic medical record.

Entity—single factor within the health system (individual hospital, clinic, or infusion center).

IS—information services.

PAR—Periodic automatic replenishment, the average or normal amount of a supply that should be kept in stock so that it does not run out prior to restocking.

Sterile services—department within the health system concerned with cleaning and sterilizing supplies.

Supply chain—department within the health system concerned with obtaining products and supplies from vendors.

System—all entities within the health system.

Considerations for Go-Live

Implementation of new pump technology is an enormous task that will impact on every discipline in the hospital or clinic. Careful coordination between departments is essential to a smooth implementation. Timing of implementation should be carefully planned. For example, the team may elect to "go-live" on intensive care units first, since the majority of pumps are used in this area. Teams that include a nurse educator, a pharmacist, and representative from biomedical engineering should arrive on the nursing unit prepared to change out pumps one by one, prepare new solutions with new tubing, change medication and solution stocks in the solution area and in the automated dispensing cabinet, and assist the nurse in programming the pump. If a change in drug concentration or solution type is incorporated into the pump go-live, electronic medical records and flowsheets will need modification. The next section includes examples of go-live checklists.

Go-Live Checklists

Implementation Team Checklist

- Develop timeline for pump rollout
- Develop contact lists for all members of the rollout team

Biomedical Services Checklist

- Clean pumps and prepare for rollout
- Attach barcodes to pumps
- Enter pumps into tracking system
- Dispose of old rental pumps, if necessary
- Determine need for new rental stock, if necessary
- Test pumps for operational functionality
- Push drug library to pumps; confirm wireless transfer
- Charge pumps for 24 hours
- Education for Biomedical staff
- Trouble-shooting tip sheets for biomedical staff
- Manufacturer test education for biomedical staff
- Education of biomedical staff on appropriate charging procedures
- Collect old pumps not in use
- Determine wireless connectivity
- Establish a storage and set-up area for pumps; verify electrical outlet or extension cord needs
- Determine process for hand-offs to sterile services

Sterile Services Checklist

- Obtain solutions needed to clean pumps
- Establish appropriate policies and procedures related to pump cleaning and storage
- Standardize supplies that will be delivered along with the pumps
- Coordinate change in supply needs to inventory manager
- Establish storage locations
- Establish PAR quantities in storage locations
- Establish procedures for medications left in the pump upon return
- Determine if new IV poles are needed
- Develop staffing schedule for rollout
- Education of staff on pump cleaning
- Determine pump charging policy when pumps not in use

Supply Chain/Inventory Specialist Checklist

- Communicate any changes in solutions and tubing (including new order numbers)
- Collaborate with pharmacy to develop a crosswalk of old solutions, new solutions, old order numbers and new order numbers
- Determine additional supplies needed for go-live teams
- Develop policies and procedures for rental pumps
- Receive and deliver pumps to the appropriate loading docks; communicate arrival with biomedical services
- Change out tubing and solutions to new products in nursing areas
- Plan for disposal or disposition of old pumps being taken out of circulation
- Update on-line ordering systems with new order numbers and PAR levels
- Order and stock new solutions
- Coordinate final delivery date of pumps
- Adjust PAR levels to meet patient care needs
- Dispose/return old tubing
- Update PAR levels in automated solution dispensing cabinets
- Update barcodes for solution shelving

Nursing/Nurse Educators

- Collaborate with implementation team and staff to develop training schedule, typically training will begin 4–6 weeks prior to implementation
- Determine staffing needs for rollout, assign super-users
- Schedule staff for training and rollout
- Develop training tools: posters, tip sheets, FAQs
- Develop tracking tool for staff education
- Upload pump network training tools to Intranet, if applicable

- Conduct training of nurses, CRNAs, nursing assistants
- Determine mode of education: should include multiple types such as class-room training, hands-on education, on-line education
- Provide education on new supplies such as tubing and solutions
- Provide trouble-shooting guides for nurses
- Support nurses on go-live day with super-users and implementation teams

Pharmacy Services Checklist

- Develop drug library content in collaboration with nursing department
- Develop drug library care areas in collaboration with nursing department
- Communicate any pharmacy process changes to nursing department
- Develop update list for any changes in automated dispensing cabinets
- Work with supply chain to determine any solution changes
- Communicate solution changes, if necessary, to all departments
- Collaborate with IS on any order set changes
- Communicate order set changes to physicians, nurses, and pharmacists
- Order new tubing supplies for the pharmacy sterile products area (IV room)
- Order new solutions, if necessary for the pharmacy department
- Develop list of changes needed in pharmacy computer systems
- Develop list of needs for bar-coding in pharmacy systems
- Develop list of changes needed in the electronic medical record, including the electronic medication administration record (MAR), flowsheets, and order sets
- Collaborate with nursing to identify any changes needed for bolus procedures (for example, if dose limits exist for boluses, there may be a change to administer bolus medications from a medication infusion bag)
- Identify any changes that may occur for medications delivered by syringe (syringe infusion pump or large volume pump syringe adaptor)
- Determine if new tubing supply will meet all medication needs, or if there are needs for alternate special tubing
- Develop list of patients on infusions on go-live day; prepare new solutions, attach new tubing; assist nurses (along with the go-live team) in changing out pumps and medication infusions. If new concentrations of infusions are used, attach warning label

Considerations for Wireless Pump Updates

Drug library updates may be frequent after the initial rollout. There may be many issues identified by nursing staff that must be addressed. There may even be mistakes in the drug library that will need correction. The implementation team's role will change; this group should identify lead individuals to participate in the maintenance phase of pump deployment. The work continues after rollout, and frequent revisions will be necessary. That said, the implementation team should identify an ideal schedule for drug library and pump updates. Constant revisions of the pump firmware or medication library is not a sustainable situation. Our team decided that, initially, we would conduct quarterly updates. As time goes on and the staff become used to the pumps, the updates can perhaps be less frequent. Chapter 11 addresses criteria for urgent pump updates compared to updates that can occur during the regularly scheduled upgrade.

There should be a process for front-line staff to request modifications to the pump library. This can be accomplished by either electronic or paper processes. When requests for changes are received, there should be a well-understood process for evaluating change requests. A multi-disciplinary team should be involved in the development of criteria for accepting drug library changes, and assigning changes to an "urgent" status versus a "non-urgent" status. Once a drug library update is accepted or a hardware or firmware upgrade is scheduled, the team will use the wireless pump update flowcharts. Individual departments should use the flowcharts, along with their go-live checklists, to make sure thorough preparations are made for any wireless pump updates.

There are some considerations for wireless pump updates that will not be included in the go-live checklists. Examples of these include:

- Maintaining an inventory of pumps that have been updated wirelessly versus those that have not been updated.
- Developing nursing policy to address expectations of nurses when updates are sent to active pumps.
- Moving pumps that are out of wireless range into wireless range so that they can receive the updates.
- Making replacement medication infusions available for pump updates, if necessary.
- Developing processes for updating any rental pumps.

Wireless Pump Update Flowcharts

Figures 13-1 through 13-3 are examples of flowcharts for wireless pump updates.

Conclusion

Wireless pump updates are complex processes that require clear accountability, and clear communication. All disciplines should have a good understanding of the processes for updates that the pump team has defined.

Request/Suggestion for Wireless Pump Updates

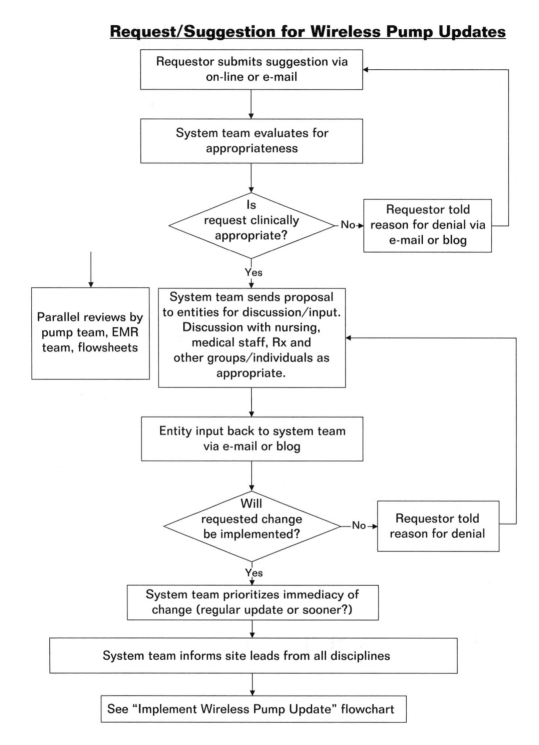

Figure 13-1. Request/suggestion for wireless pump updates.

Implement Wireless Pump Change

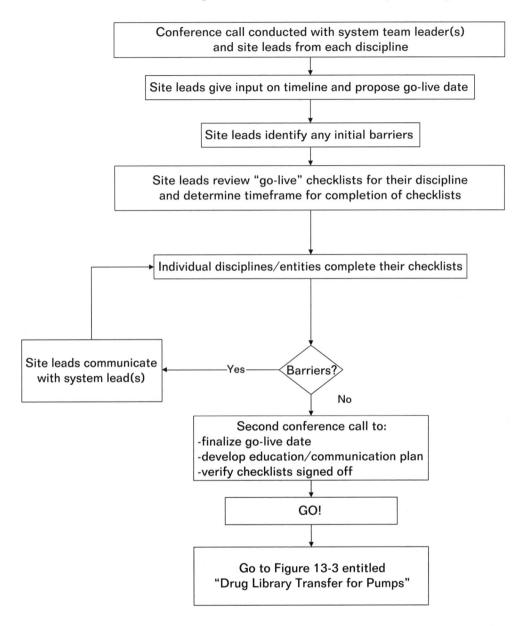

Figure 13-2. Implement wireless pump change.

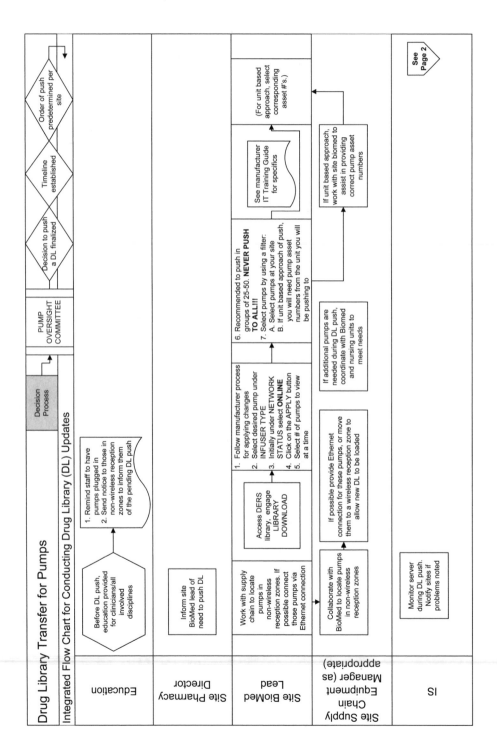

Figure 13-3. Drug library transfer for pumps.

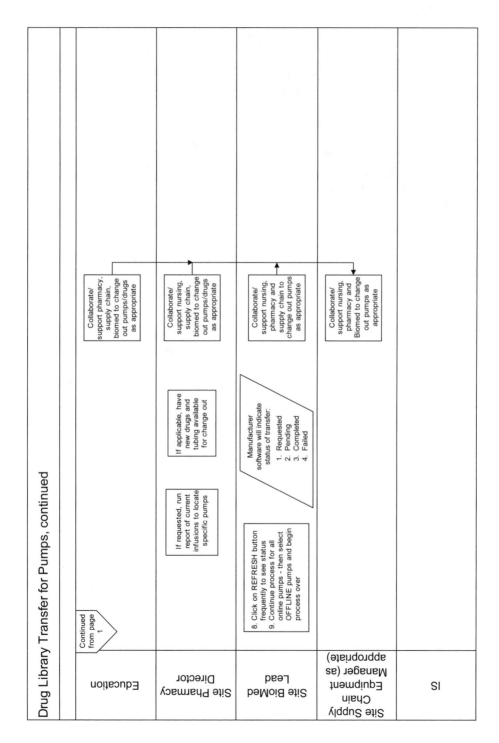

Figure 13-3 (cont'd). Drug library transfer for pumps.

PRACTICE TIPS

- Plan ahead for pump updates: identify a lead group to manage the pump and library upgrades.
- Identify approval process for pump library changes; make checklists for each department, so that no step is overlooked.
- Identify the impact of pump library changes on the electronic medical record, the eMAR, the flowsheets, and any order sets.
- Pump tracking is essential during a pump library update; you will need to be able to track which pumps have the new library or software on them, and which have the old version.
- Identify a team of pharmacists and nurses to conduct the pump "swap." This may include the preparation of new infusion bags.
- Practicing a "dry run" of library or software updates ahead of time will identify any issues and challenges in the updates.

Suggested Reading

Aston G. Pump up your data; tracking smart pump trends can boost safety, outcomes. Materials Management in Healthcare 2009. Available at: www.matmanmag.com Accessed April 29, 2009.

Sanborn M, Cohen T. Get smart: effective use of smart pump technology. *Hosp Pharm.* 2009;44;348-353.

Wetterneck TB, Skibinski KA, Roberts TL, et al. Using failure mode and effects analysis to plan implementation of smart i.v. pump technology. *Am J Health-Syst Pharm.* 2006;63:1528-1538.

Disclaimer: This information is provided for demonstration purposes only. ASHP makes no representations about the validity, accuracy, reliability or suitability of the information, specifically disclaims liability for consequences that may arise in connection with the information, and urges practitioners to exercise their best professional judgments about the dosing limits presented. Dosing limits should be based upon hospital utilization patterns, as well as on acceptable dosing ranges. Practitioners are advised that some of the dosing limits presented here may exceed FDA-approved doses. This was done to avoid excessive alerts and alert fatigue. Practitioners are advised to use caution when determining appropriate dosing limits.

Table A-1. Continuous Dosing

Displayed Name	CCA Name	Med. Amount	Med. Unit	Diluent Amount	Diluent Unit
aminocaproic acid	ICU	5	grams	100	mL
AMIODarone	ICU	500	mg	500	mL
AMIODarone	ICU	1500	mg	250	mL
cisatracurium	ICU	200	mg	100	mL
dexmedetomidine	ICU	200	mcg	50	mL
dexmedetomidine	ICU	400	mcg	100	mL
DOBUTamine	ICU	500	mg	250	mL
DOBUTamine	ICU	1000	mg	250	mL
DOPamine	ICU	400	mg	250	mL
DOPamine	ICU	800	mg	250	mL
EPInephrine	ICU	5	mg	250	mL
EPInephrine	ICU	16	mg	250	mL
EPInephrine-mcg/kg/min dosing	ICU	5	mg	250	mL
EPInephrine-mcg/kg/min dosing	ICU	16	mg	250	mL
esmolol	ICU	2000	mg	100	mL
HEParin	ICU	25000	units	250	mL
isoproterenol	ICU	1	mg	50	mL
isoproterenol-mcg/kg/min dosing	ICU	1	mg	50	mL
lidocaine	ICU	2	grams	250	mL
milrinone	ICU	20	mg	100	mL
NICARdipine	ICU	25	mg	250	mL
NICARdipine	ICU	100	mg	250	mL
nitroGLYCERIN	ICU	50	mg	250	mL
nitroGLYCERIN	ICU	200	mg	250	mL
nitroGLYCERIN-mcg/kg/min dosing	ICU	50	mg	250	mL
nitroGLYCERIN-mcg/kg/min dosing	ICU	200	mg	250	mL
nitroPRUSSide	ICU	100	mg	250	mL
nitroPRUSSide	ICU	400	mg	250	mL
NOREPInephrine	ICU	8	mg	250	mL
NOREPInephrine	ICU	16	mg	250	mL
NOREPInephrine-mcg/kg/min dosing	ICU	8	mg	250	mL
NOREPInephrine-mcg/kg/min dosing	ICU	16	mg	250	mL
phenylephrine	ICU	50	mg	250	mL

Source: With permission from Fairview Health Services, Minneapolis, Minnesota.

Med. Max. Rate	Dose Rate Dosing Unit	Dose Rate LHL	Dose Rate LSL	Dose Rate USL	Dose Rate UHL
	grams/hr			5	
	mg/min		0.4		2
	mg/min		0.4		2
	mcg/kg/min		0.2	15	20
	mcg/kg/hr		0.2	0.8	1.3
	mcg/kg/hr		0.2	0.8	1.3
	mcg/kg/min			20	
	mcg/kg/min			20	
	mcg/kg/min		1	20	
	mcg/kg/min		1	20	
	mcg/min		0.5	15	
	mcg/min		0.5	15	
	mcg/kg/min		0.01	0.5	
	mcg/kg/min		0.01	0.5	
	mcg/kg/min			300	350
	units/hr	50	200	2000	2500
	mcg/min		0.09	20	
	mcg/kg/min		0.01	0.3	
	mg/min		0.5	4	6
	mcg/kg/min		0.1		1
	mg/hr		4	16	
	mg/hr		4	16	
	mcg/min		1.5	200	
	mcg/min		1.5	200	
	mcg/kg/min		0.05	3	
	mcg/kg/min		0.05	3	
	mcg/kg/min		0.1	5	10
	mcg/kg/min		0.1	5	10
	mcg/min		1	99	
	mcg/min		1	99	
	mcg/kg/min		0.02	0.9	
	mcg/kg/min		0.02	0.9	
	mcg/min		5	250	

Source: With permission from Fairview Health Services, Minneapolis, Minnesota.

Table A-1. Continuous Dosing (cont'd)

Displayed Name	CCA Name	Med. Amount	Med. Unit	Diluent Amount	Diluent Unit
phenylephrine-mcg/kg/min dosing	ICU	50	mg	250	mL
phenylephrine-mcg/kg/min dosing	ICU	200	mg	250	mL
propofol	ICU	1000	mg	100	mL
vasopressin	ICU	100	units	100	mL
vecuronium	ICU	50	mg	50	mL
IV fluid	ICU				mL
23.4% Sodium Chloride	ICU			30	mL
3% sodium chloride	ICU				mL
abciximab less than 80 kg	ICU	9	mg	250	mL
abciximab 80 kg or more	ICU	9	mg	250	mL
acetylcysteine Step 1	ICU		grams	200	mL
acetylcysteine Step 2	ICU		grams	500	mL
acetylcysteine Step 3	ICU		grams	1000	mL
acetylcysteine-renal	ICU	600	mg	100	mL
acetylcysteine-renal	ICU	1200	mg	100	mL
alemtuzumab	ICU		mg	100	mL
alprostadil	ICU	1	mg	100	mL
alteplase PE	ICU	100	mg	100	mL
alteplase-rad	ICU	1	mg	100	mL
alteplase stroke	ICU		mg		mL
antibiotic (except vancomycin)	ICU			50	mL
antibiotic (except vancomycin)	ICU			100	mL
antibiotic (except vancomycin)	ICU			150	mL
antibiotic (except vancomycin)	ICU			250	mL
antibiotic (except vancomycin)	ICU			500	mL
antithymocyte globulin horse	ICU		mg	50	mL
antithymocyte globulin horse	ICU		mg	100	mL
antithymocyte globulin horse	ICU		mg	150	mL
antithymocyte globulin horse	ICU		grams	250	mL
antithymocyte globulin horse	ICU		grams	500	mL
argatroban non-cath lab	ICU	250	mg	250	mL
argatroban-cath lab	ICU	250	mg	250	mL
basiliximab	ICU		mg	50	mL
BEVACizumab over 30 min	ICU		mg	100	mL
BEVACizumab over 60 min	ICU		mg	100	mL

Source: With permission from Fairview Health Services, Minneapolis, Minnesota.

Med. Max. Rate	Dose Rate Dosing Unit	Dose Rate LHL	Dose Rate LSL	Dose Rate USL	Dose Rate UHL
	mcg/kg/min		0.2	3	
	mcg/kg/min		0.2	3	
	mcg/kg/min		4	200	300
	units/hr	0.1	0.5	2.5	10
	mcg/kg/min		0.2	2	3
	mL/hr				1000
	mL/hr			120	180
	mL/hr				100
	mcg/kg/min				0.125
	mcg/min		5		10
	mL/hr				200
	mL/hr				125
	mL/hr				62.5
	mL/hr			400	
	mL/hr			400	
	mL/hr			80	
	mcg/kg/min			0.15	0.4
	mg/hr		50	50	100
	mg/hr	0.1	0.24	1	2
	mg/hr				81
	mL/hr		25	300	
	mL/hr		50	400	
	mL/hr		75	150	
	mL/hr		125	250	
	mL/hr		100	500	
	mL/hr			20	
	mL/hr			40	
	mL/hr			52	
	mL/hr			80	
	mL/hr			155	
	mcg/kg/min			5	10
	mcg/kg/min			30	40
	mL/hr		50		150
	mL/hr			320	
	mL/hr			160	

Source: With permission from Fairview Health Services, Minneapolis, Minnesota.

Table A-1. Continuous Dosing (cont'd)

Displayed Name	CCA Name	Med. Amount	Med. Unit	Diluent Amount	Diluent Unit
BEVACizumab over 90 min	ICU		mg	100	mL
bivalirudin non-cath lab	ICU	250	mg	50	mL
bivalirudin-cath lab	ICU	250	mg	50	mL
bumetanide ICU	ICU	25	mg	100	mL
calcium CHLORide	ICU		grams	100	mL
calcium GLUConate	ICU	1	grams	100	mL
chlorpromazine	ICU	25	mg	50	mL
chlorpromazine	ICU	50	mg	100	mL
cidofovir	ICU		mg	100	mL
clevidipine	ICU	25	mg	50	mL
conivaptan	ICU	20	mg	250	mL
cyclosporine	ICU		mg	100	mL
cyclosporine	ICU		mg	150	mL
cyclosporine	ICU		mg	250	mL
cyclosporine drip BMT	ICU	250	mg	250	mL
cyclosporine drip BMT	ICU	500	mg	250	mL
cyclosporine drip-solid organ	ICU	250	mg	250	mL
cyclosporine drip-solid organ	ICU	500	mg	250	mL
daclizumab	ICU		mg	50	mL
dantrolene	ICU		mg		mL
deferoxamine	ICU		mg	250	mL
desmopressin	ICU		mcg	50	mL
echo-DOBUTamine	ICU	500	mg	250	mL
diltiazem	ICU	125	mg	125	mL
drotrecogin alfa (xigris)	ICU	10	mg	100	mL
drotrecogin alfa (xigris)	ICU	20	mg	200	mL
eptifibatide	ICU	200	mg	100	mL
fentanyl	ICU	5	mg	100	mL
ferric gluconate	ICU	125	mg	100	mL
ferric gluconate	ICU	250	mg	250	mL
foscarnet	ICU		mg		mL
fosphenytoin	ICU		mg		mL
furosemide	ICU	100	mg	100	mL
ganciclovir	ICU		mg	100	mL
HYDROmorphone	ICU		mg		mL
immune globulin-sucrose	ICU				mL
immune globulin-sucrose free	ICU				mL

Source: With permission from Fairview Health Services, Minneapolis, Minnesota.

Med. Max. Rate	Dose Rate Dosing Unit	Dose Rate LHL	Dose Rate LSL	Dose Rate USL	Dose Rate UHL
	mL/hr			107	
	mg/kg/hr	0.19			0.2
	mg/kg/hr				1.75
	mg/hr		0.5		4
	grams/hr				4
	grams/hr				4
	mL/hr			100	
	mL/hr			100	
	mL/hr			115	130
	mg/hr			32	
	mg/hr	0.8			1.7
	mL/hr				80
	mL/hr				105
	mL/hr				160
	mg/hr			16	20
	mg/hr			16	20
	mg/hr			5	9.9
	mg/hr			5	9.9
	mL/hr			210	
	mg/hr			500	
	mg/hr			1500	
	mL/hr			200	
	mcg/kg/min			100	
	mg/hr		1	15	20
	mcg/kg/hr	0.5	23.9		24
	mcg/kg/hr	0.5	23.9		24
	mcg/kg/min				2
	mcg/hr				
	mL/hr				120
	mL/hr				150
	mL/hr			500	
	mg/min				150
	mg/hr			30	60
	mL/hr			160	
	mg/hr				
	mL/kg/hr		0.5		2.5
	mL/kg/hr		0.5		4

Source: With permission from Fairview Health Services, Minneapolis, Minnesota.

Table A-1. Continuous Dosing (cont'd)

Displayed Name	CCA Name	Med. Amount	Med. Unit	Diluent Amount	Diluent Unit
infliximab	ICU		mg	250	mL
insulin-ICU	ICU	50	units	50	mL
iron dextran test dose	ICU	25	mg	50	mL
iron dextran	ICU		mg	500	mL
iron sucrose (Venofer)	ICU	200	mg	100	mL
iron sucrose (Venofer)	ICU	500	mg	250	mL
ketamine	ICU		mg		mL
labetalol	ICU	250	mg	50	mL
lepirudin	ICU	100	mg	250	mL
leucovorin	ICU	10	mg	1	mL
levetiracetam	ICU			100	mL
lipids 20%	ICU	50	grams	250	mL
lipids anesthetic overdose	ICU	50	grams	250	mL
lorazepam	ICU	50	mg	50	mL
lorazepam	ICU	100	mg	100	mL
magnesium replacement	ICU		grams		mL
methylprednisolone	ICU		mg	100	mL
methylpred INF spinal cord	ICU		mg	500	mL
methylpred bolus spinal cord	ICU		mg	100	mL
metoclopramide	ICU		mg	50	mL
midazolam	ICU	100	mg	100	mL
morphine	ICU		mg		mL
mycophenolate 500 mg dose	ICU	500	mg		mL
mycophenolate 1000 mg dose	ICU	1000	mg		mL
mycophenolate 1500 mg dose	ICU	1500	mg		mL
naloxone	ICU	4	mg	100	mL
nesiritide	ICU	1.5	mg	250	mL
octreotide	ICU	1250	mcg	250	mL
ondansetron drip	ICU	50	mg	50	mL
Other Drug	ICU		Select on In-fuser		mL
PANtoprazole	ICU	80	mg	100	mL
PenTobarbital	ICU	2000	mg	250	mL
PHenobarbital	ICU	2000	mg	250	mL
phenytoin	ICU		mg		mL
phytonadione (vitamin K)	ICU		mg	50	mL

Source: With permission from Fairview Health Services, Minneapolis, Minnesota.

Med. Max. Rate	Dose Rate Dosing Unit	Dose Rate LHL	Dose Rate LSL	Dose Rate USL	Dose Rate UHL
	mL/hr		120	126	130
	units/hr		0.5	20	80
	mL/hr				200
	mL/hr		62.5	84	100
	mL/hr				120
	mL/hr			62.5	75
	mg/hr				20
	mg/min		0.1	6	10
	mg/kg/hr		0.02	0.21	
	mg/min				160
	mL/hr			400	
	mL/hr		1	25	62.5
	mL/hr		750	1000	
	mg/hr		0.2	20	30
	mg/hr		0.2	20	30
	grams/hr				2
	mL/hr				400
	mg/kg/hr				5.4
	mL/hr				400
	mL/hr				200
	mg/hr		0.2	20	30
	mg/hr				
	mg/hr				250
	mg/hr				500
	mg/hr				750
	mg/hr		0.05	1	
	mcg/kg/min		0.005		0.03
	mcg/hr			150	250
	mg/hr				5
	mg/hr		7.9		8
	mg/kg/hr		0.1	3	5
	mg/hr			15	
	mg/min	1	5	35	50
	mL/hr				100

Source: With permission from Fairview Health Services, Minneapolis, Minnesota.

Table A-1. Continuous Dosing (cont'd)

Displayed Name	CCA Name	Med. Amount	Med. Unit	Diluent Amount	Diluent Unit
potassium chloride	ICU	10	mEq	100	mL
potassium chloride	ICU	20	mEq	50	mL
potassium phosphate	ICU		mmol	250	mL
potassium phosphate	ICU		mmol	500	mL
procainamide	ICU	2	grams	250	mL
rituximab	ICU	1	mg	1	mL
rocuronium	ICU	500	mg	250	mL
sodium bicarbonate	ICU		mEq		mL
sodium phosphate	ICU		mmol	250	mL
sodium phosphate	ICU		mmol	500	mL
tacrolimus	ICU	5	mg	250	mL
tenecteplase	ICU	5	mg	500	mL
thymoglobulin	ICU	50	mg	115	mL
thymoglobulin	ICU	75	mg	173	mL
thymoglobulin	ICU	100	mg	283	mL
thymoglobulin-peripheral	ICU		mg	500	mL
TPN	ICU				mL
valproate	ICU		mg	100	mL
vancomycin	ICU		mg		mL
zoledronic acid	ICU		mg	100	mL
IV fluid	MedSurg				mL
blood products	MedSurg				mL
antibiotic (except vancomycin)	MedSurg			50	mL
antibiotic (except vancomycin)	MedSurg			100	mL
antibiotic (except vancomycin)	MedSurg			150	mL
antibiotic (except vancomycin)	MedSurg			250	mL
antibiotic (except vancomycin)	MedSurg			500	mL
vancomycin	MedSurg		mg		mL
potassium chloride	MedSurg	10	mEq	100	mL
potassium chloride	MedSurg	20	mEq	50	mL
magnesium replacement	MedSurg		grams		mL
TPN	MedSurg				mL
lipids 20%	MedSurg	50	grams	250	mL
lipids 20%	MedSurg	100	grams	500	mL
HEParin	MedSurg	25000	units	250	mL
acetylcysteine-renal	MedSurg	600	mg	100	mL
acetylcysteine-renal	MedSurg	1200	mg	100	mL

Source: With permission from Fairview Health Services, Minneapolis, Minnesota.

Med. Max. Rate	Dose Rate Dosing Unit	Dose Rate LHL	Dose Rate LSL	Dose Rate USL	Dose Rate UHL
	mEq/hr				10
	mEq/hr			20	40
	mL/hr			65	86
	mL/hr			86	125
	mg/min		0.5	4	6
	mL/hr				400
	mcg/kg/min		4	16	
	mEq/hr			50	
	mL/hr			65	86
	mL/hr			86	125
	mcg/hr	5	10	120	200
	mg/hr	0.05	0.1	1	1.2
	mL/hr			29	
	mL/hr			44	
	mL/hr			71	
	mL/hr			135	
	mL/hr			250	300
	mL/hr			100	
	mg/hr			1700	2500
	mL/hr				460
	mL/hr				1000
	mL/hr				1000
	mL/hr		25	300	
	mL/hr		50	400	
	mL/hr		75	150	
	mL/hr		125	250	
	mL/hr		100	500	
	mg/hr			1700	2500
	mEq/hr				10
	mEq/hr			20	40
	grams/hr				2
	mL/hr			250	300
	mL/hr		1	25	62.5
	mL/hr		1	25	62.5
	units/hr	50	200	2000	2500
	mL/hr			400	
	mL/hr			400	

Source: With permission from Fairview Health Services, Minneapolis, Minnesota.

Table A-1. Continuous Dosing (cont'd)

Displayed Name	CCA Name	Med. Amount	Med. Unit	Diluent Amount	Diluent Unit
alemtuzumab	MedSurg		mg	100	mL
alteplase stroke	MedSurg		mg		mL
alteplase PE	MedSurg	100	mg	100	mL
alteplase-rad	MedSurg	12.5	mg	50	mL
AMIODarone	MedSurg	500	mg	500	mL
argatroban non-cath lab	MedSurg	250	mg	250	mL
basiliximab	MedSurg		mg	50	mL
BEVACizumab over 30 min	MedSurg		mg	100	mL
BEVACizumab over 60 min	MedSurg		mg	100	mL
BEVACizumab over 90 min	MedSurg		mg	100	mL
bumetanide	MedSurg	25	mg	100	mL
calcium CHLORide	MedSurg		grams	100	mL
calcium GLUConate	MedSurg	1	grams	100	mL
chlorpromazine	MedSurg	25	mg	50	mL
chlorpromazine	MedSurg	50	mg	100	mL
conivaptan	MedSurg	20	mg	250	mL
cyclosporine drip-solid organ	MedSurg	250	mg	250	mL
cyclosporine drip-solid organ	MedSurg	500	mg	250	mL
daclizumab	MedSurg		mg	50	mL
deferoxamine	MedSurg		mg	250	mL
desmopressin	MedSurg		mcg	50	mL
diltiazem	MedSurg	125	mg	125	mL
ferric gluconate	MedSurg	125	mg	100	mL
ferric gluconate	MedSurg	250	mg	250	mL
foscarnet	MedSurg		mg		mL
fosphenytoin	MedSurg		mg		mL
furosemide	MedSurg	100	mg	100	mL
ganciclovir	MedSurg		mg	100	mL
immune globulin-sucrose	MedSurg				mL
immune globulin-sucrose free	MedSurg				mL
infliximab	MedSurg		mg	250	mL
insulin	MedSurg	50	units	50	mL
iron dextran test dose	MedSurg	25	mg	50	mL
iron dextran	MedSurg		mg	500	mL
iron sucrose (Venofer)	MedSurg	200	mg	100	mL
iron sucrose (Venofer)	MedSurg	500	mg	250	mL
lepirudin	MedSurg	100	mg	250	mL

Source: With permission from Fairview Health Services, Minneapolis, Minnesota.

Med. Max. Rate	Dose Rate Dosing Unit	Dose Rate LHL	Dose Rate LSL	Dose Rate USL	Dose Rate UHL
	mL/hr			80	
	mg/hr				81
	mg/hr		50	50	100
	mg/hr	0.1	0.24		2
	mg/min		0.4		2
	mcg/kg/min			5	10
	mL/hr		50		150
	mL/hr			320	
	mL/hr			160	
	mL/hr			107	
	mg/hr		0.5		2
	grams/hr				4
	grams/hr				4
	mL/hr			100	
	mL/hr			100	
	mg/hr	0.8			1.7
	mg/hr			5	9.9
	mg/hr			5	9.9
	mL/hr			210	
	mg/hr			1500	
	mL/hr			200	
	mg/hr		1	15	20
	mL/hr				120
	mL/hr				150
	mL/hr			500	
	mg/min				150
	mg/hr			30	60
	mL/hr			160	
	mL/kg/hr		0.5		2.5
	mL/kg/hr		0.5		4
	mL/hr		120	126	130
	units/hr		0.5	10	30
	mL/hr				200
	mL/hr		62.5	84	100
	mL/hr				120
	mL/hr			62.5	75
	mg/kg/hr		0.02	0.21	

Source: With permission from Fairview Health Services, Minneapolis, Minnesota.

Table A-1. Continuous Dosing (cont'd)

Displayed Name	CCA Name	Med. Amount	Med. Unit	Diluent Amount	Diluent Unit
levetiracetam	MedSurg			100	mL
mannitol injection 20%	MedSurg	50	grams	250	mL
mannitol injection 20%	MedSurg	100	grams	500	mL
mannitol injection 25%	MedSurg	12.5	grams	50	mL
mannitol injection 25%	MedSurg		grams		mL
metoclopramide	MedSurg		mg	50	mL
methylprednisolone	MedSurg		mg	100	mL
mycophenolate 500 mg dose	MedSurg	500	mg		mL
mycophenolate 1000 mg dose	MedSurg	1000	mg		mL
mycophenolate 1500 mg dose	MedSurg	1500	mg		mL
naloxone	MedSurg	4	mg	100	mL
octreotide	MedSurg	1250	mcg	250	mL
ondansetron drip	MedSurg	50	mg	50	mL
Other Drug	MedSurg		Select on Infuser		mL
PANtoprazole	MedSurg	80	mg	100	mL
phytonadione (vitamin K)	MedSurg		mg	50	mL
potassium phosphate	MedSurg		mmol	250	mL
potassium phosphate	MedSurg		mmol	500	mL
rituximab	MedSurg	1	mg	1	mL
sodium bicarbonate	MedSurg		mEq		mL
1.5% sodium chloride	MedSurg			1000	mL
3% sodium chloride	MedSurg				mL
sodium phosphate	MedSurg		mmol	250	mL
sodium phosphate	MedSurg		mmol	500	mL
tacrolimus	MedSurg	5	mg	250	mL
thymoglobulin	MedSurg	50	mg	115	mL
thymoglobulin	MedSurg	75	mg	173	mL
thymoglobulin	MedSurg	100	mg	283	mL
thymoglobulin-peripheral	MedSurg		mg	500	mL
valproate	MedSurg		mg	100	mL
IV fluid	OB				mL
oxytocin-labor	OB	20	units	1000	mL
oxytocin-postpartum	OB	20	units	1000	mL
oxytocin-postpartum	OB	40	units	1000	mL
magnesium sulfate infusion	OB	20	grams	500	mL

Source: With permission from Fairview Health Services, Minneapolis, Minnesota.

Med. Max. Rate	Dose Rate Dosing Unit	Dose Rate LHL	Dose Rate LSL	Dose Rate USL	Dose Rate UHL
	mL/hr			400	
	mL/hr			1000	
	mL/hr			1000	
	mL/hr			1000	
	mL/hr			1000	
	mL/hr				200
	mL/hr				400
	mg/hr				250
	mg/hr				500
	mg/hr				750
	mg/hr		0.05	1	
	mcg/hr			150	250
	mg/hr				5
	mg/hr		7.9		8
	mL/hr				100
	mL/hr			65	86
	mL/hr			86	125
	mL/hr				400
	mEq/hr			50	
	mL/hr			500	
	mL/hr				100
	mL/hr			65	86
	mL/hr			86	125
	mcg/hr	5	10	120	200
	mL/hr			29	
	mL/hr			44	
	mL/hr			71	
	mL/hr			135	
	mL/hr			100	
	mL/hr				1000
	milliUnits/min			24	40
	mL/hr			125	
	mL/hr			125	
	grams/hr	0.2	0.5	4	6

Source: With permission from Fairview Health Services, Minneapolis, Minnesota.

Table A-1. Continuous Dosing (cont'd)

Displayed Name	CCA Name	Med. Amount	Med. Unit	Diluent Amount	Diluent Unit
magnesium seizure	OB	2	grams	50	mL
magnesium seizure	OB	4	grams	50	mL
antibiotic (except vancomycin)	OB			50	mL
antibiotic (except vancomycin)	OB			100	mL
antibiotic (except vancomycin)	OB			150	mL
antibiotic (except vancomycin)	OB			250	mL
antibiotic (except vancomycin)	OB			500	mL
vancomycin	OB		mg		mL
blood products	OB				mL
HEParin	OB	25000	units	250	mL
insulin-OB	OB	50	units	50	mL
TPN	OB				mL
lipids 20%	OB	50	grams	250	mL
lipids 20%	OB	100	grams	500	mL
potassium chloride	OB	10	mEq	100	mL
hetastarch (Hespan)	OB			500	mL
Other Drug	OB		Select on Infuser		mL
fosphenytoin	OB		mg		mL
zidovudine	OB		mg		mL
IV fluid	Oncology				mL
premedication	Oncology		mg	50	mL
premedication	Oncology		mg	100	mL
premedication	Oncology		mg	150	mL
ALDESleukin	Oncology		Million Units	50	mL
alemtuzumab	Oncology		mg	100	mL
amifostine	Oncology		mg	50	mL
antithymocyte globulin horse	Oncology		mg	50	mL
antithymocyte globulin horse	Oncology		mg	100	mL
antithymocyte globulin horse	Oncology		mg	150	mL
antithymocyte globulin horse	Oncology		grams	250	mL
antithymocyte globulin horse	Oncology		grams	500	mL
arsenic trioxide	Oncology		mg	250	mL
L-asparaginase	Oncology		units	50	mL
azacitidine	Oncology		mg	100	mL
bendamustine	Oncology		mg	500	mL

Source: With permission from Fairview Health Services, Minneapolis, Minnesota.

Med. Max. Rate	Dose Rate Dosing Unit	Dose Rate LHL	Dose Rate LSL	Dose Rate USL	Dose Rate UHL
	mL/hr				600
	mL/hr				200
	mL/hr		25	300	
	mL/hr		50	400	
	mL/hr		75	150	
	mL/hr		125	250	
	mL/hr		100	500	
	mg/hr			1700	2500
	mL/hr				1000
	units/hr	50	200	2000	2500
	units/hr		0.3	3	5
	mL/hr			250	300
	mL/hr		1	25	62.5
	mL/hr		1	25	62.5
	mEq/hr				10
	mL/hr				1000
	mg/min				150
	mg/kg/hr			1	
	mL/hr				1000
	mL/hr				250
	mL/hr				400
	mL/hr				600
	mL/hr			300	
	mL/hr			80	
	mL/hr			300	
	mL/hr			20	
	mL/hr			40	
	mL/hr			52	
	mL/hr			80	
	mL/hr			155	
	mL/hr			320	
	mL/hr			58	
	mL/hr			240	
	mL/hr			1000	

Source: With permission from Fairview Health Services, Minneapolis, Minnesota.

Table A-1. Continuous Dosing (cont'd)

Displayed Name	CCA Name	Med. Amount	Med. Unit	Diluent Amount	Diluent Unit
BEVACizumab over 30 min	Oncology		mg	100	mL
BEVACizumab over 60 min	Oncology		mg	100	mL
BEVACizumab over 90 min	Oncology		mg	100	mL
bleomycin	Oncology		units	50	mL
busulfan	Oncology	0.5	mg	1	mL
CARBoplatin	Oncology		mg	100	mL
CARBoplatin	Oncology		mg	250	mL
CARBoplatin	Oncology		mg	500	mL
CARBoplatin over 24 hr	Oncology		mg	1000	mL
CARBoplatin desens	Oncology		mg	100	mL
CARBoplatin desens	Oncology		mg	150	mL
carmustine (BCNU)	Oncology		mg	250	mL
CETuximab	Oncology	2	mg	1	mL
chemotherapy infusion	Oncology				mL
CISplatin	Oncology		mg	250	mL
CISplatin	Oncology		mg	500	mL
CISplatin	Oncology		mg	1000	mL
CISplatin NO manitol	Oncology	1	mg	1	mL
cladribine	Oncology		mg	250	mL
clofarabine	Oncology	0.4	mg	1	mL
cycloPHOSPHAMIDE	Oncology		mg	250	mL
cycloPHOSPHAMIDE	Oncology		mg	500	mL
CYTarabine (high dose)	Oncology		grams	250	mL
CYTarabine over 1 hr	Oncology		mg	100	mL
CYTarabine over 3 hrs	Oncology		mg	250	mL
CYTarabine continuous infusion	Oncology		mg	1000	mL
dacarbazine	Oncology		mg	250	mL
DAUNOrubicin	Oncology		mg	100	mL
DAUNOrubicin liposomal	Oncology	1	mg	1	mL
decitabine	Oncology		mg	100	mL
decitabine	Oncology		mg	250	mL
dexrazoxane (Totect)	Oncology		mg	1000	mL
dexrazoxane (Zinecard)	Oncology		mg	100	mL
DOCetaxel	Oncology		mg	250	mL
DOCetaxel	Oncology		mg	500	mL
DOXOrubicin over 1 hr	Oncology		mg	100	mL
DOXOrubicin over 24 hr	Oncology		mg	1000	mL

Source: With permission from Fairview Health Services, Minneapolis, Minnesota.

Med. Max. Rate	Dose Rate Dosing Unit	Dose Rate LHL	Dose Rate LSL	Dose Rate USL	Dose Rate UHL
	mL/hr			320	
	mL/hr			160	
	mL/hr			107	
	mL/hr			300	
	mg/kg/hr			0.45	
	mL/hr			240	
	mL/hr			470	
	mL/hr			1000	
	mL/hr			50	
	mL/hr			100	
	mL/hr			150	
	mL/hr			320	
	mL/hr				300
	mL/hr				
	mL/hr			320	
	mL/hr			610	
	mL/hr			1000	
	mg/min			1	
	mL/hr			160	
	mL/hr			75	
	mL/hr			640	
	mL/hr			1000	
	mL/hr			320	
	mL/hr			160	
	mL/hr			110	
	mL/hr			50	
	mL/hr			640	
	mL/hr			320	
	mL/hr			140	
	mL/hr			160	
	mL/hr			320	
	mL/hr			1000	
	mL/hr			640	
	mL/hr			320	
	mL/hr			610	
	mL/hr			160	
	mL/hr			50	

Source: With permission from Fairview Health Services, Minneapolis, Minnesota.

Table A-1. Continuous Dosing (cont'd)

Displayed Name	CCA Name	Med. Amount	Med. Unit	Diluent Amount	Diluent Unit
DOXOrubicin liposomal	Oncology		mg	250	mL
DOXOrubicin liposomal	Oncology		mg	500	mL
eculizumab	Oncology	600	mg	120	mL
eculizumab	Oncology	900	mg	180	mL
etoposide VP-16	Oncology		mg	250	mL
etoposide VP-16	Oncology		mg	500	mL
etoposide VP-16	Oncology		mg	1000	mL
etoposide phosphate (Etopophos)	Oncology		mg	100	mL
floxuridine	Oncology		mg	500	mL
FLUdarabine	Oncology		mg	100	mL
fluorouracil over 24 hrs	Oncology		mg	1000	mL
ganciclovir	Oncology		mg	100	mL
gemcitabine	Oncology		grams	250	mL
gemtuzumab	Oncology		mg	100	mL
IDArubicin	Oncology		mg	100	mL
ifosfamide	Oncology		grams	100	mL
ifosfamide	Oncology		grams	250	mL
ifosfamide	Oncology		grams	1000	mL
ifosfamide + mesna	Oncology			1000	mL
interferon alpha	Oncology		units	100	mL
investigational chemo	Oncology		mg		mL
irinotecan	Oncology		mg	250	mL
irinotecan	Oncology		mg	500	mL
ixabepilone	Oncology		mg	250	mL
mesna intermittent	Oncology		mg	50	mL
mesna cont infusion	Oncology		mg	1000	mL
METHOTREXate/sodium Bicarb	Oncology			500	mL
METHOTREXate/sodium bicarb	Oncology			1000	mL
METHOTREXate	Oncology		mg	100	mL
mitoxantrone	Oncology		mg	50	mL
natalizumab	Oncology	300	mg	100	mL
nelarabine	Oncology	5	mg	1	mL
Other Drug	Oncology		Select on Infuser		mL
oxaliplatin	Oncology		mg	500	mL
PACLitaxel over 1 hour	Oncology		mg	250	mL

Source: With permission from Fairview Health Services, Minneapolis, Minnesota.

Med. Max. Rate	Dose Rate Dosing Unit	Dose Rate LHL	Dose Rate LSL	Dose Rate USL	Dose Rate UHL
	mL/hr			320	
	mL/hr			610	
	mL/hr			240	
	mL/hr			360	
	mL/hr			640	
	mL/hr			610	
	mL/hr			1000	
	mL/hr			160	
	mL/hr			610	
	mL/hr			320	
	mL/hr				50
	mL/hr			160	
	mL/hr			640	
	mL/hr			80	
	mL/hr			640	
	mL/hr			320	
	mL/hr			640	
	mL/hr			385	
	mL/hr			60	
	mL/hr			350	
	mL/hr				
	mL/hr			320	
	mL/hr			610	
	mL/hr			110	
	mL/hr			300	
	mL/hr			60	
	mL/hr			150	
	mL/hr			290	
	mL/hr			320	
	mL/hr			105	
	mg/hr			300	
	mL/hr			600	
	mL/hr			320	
	mL/hr			320	

Source: With permission from Fairview Health Services, Minneapolis, Minnesota.

Table A-1. Continuous Dosing (cont'd)

Displayed Name	CCA Name	Med. Amount	Med. Unit	Diluent Amount	Diluent Unit
PACLitaxel over 3 hours	Oncology		mg	500	mL
PACLitaxel over 24 hours	Oncology		mg	500	mL
PACLitaxel prtn bd (abraxane)	Oncology	5	mg	1	mL
pegaspargase	Oncology		units	100	mL
pemetrexed	Oncology		mg	100	mL
pentostatin	Oncology		mg	50	mL
rasburicase	Oncology		mg	50	mL
rituximab	Oncology	1	mg	1	mL
streptozocin	Oncology		mg	100	mL
TEMSIRolimus	Oncology		mg	250	mL
teniposide	Oncology		mg	250	mL
teniposide	Oncology		mg	500	mL
teniposide	Oncology		mg	1000	mL
thiotepa	Oncology		mg	50	mL
thiotepa	Oncology		mg	100	mL
thiotepa	Oncology		mg	250	mL
topotecan	Oncology		mg	100	mL
TRASTuzumab over 30 min	Oncology		mg	250	mL
TRASTuzumab over 90 min	Oncology		mg	250	mL
vinBLAStine-infuse via gravity	Oncology		mg	25	mL
vinCRISTine	Oncology		mg	1000	mL
vinCRIStine infuse via gravity	Oncology		mg	25	mL
vinoRELBine infuse via gravity	Oncology		mg	25	mL
zoledronic acid	Oncology		mg	100	mL
IV fluid	Outpt Infu				mL
Premedication	Outpt Infu		mg		mL
blood products	Outpt Infu				mL
potassium chloride	Outpt Infu	10	mEq	100	mL
potassium chloride	Outpt Infu	20	mEq	50	mL
magnesium replacement	Outpt Infu	1	grams	50	mL
magnesium replacement	Outpt Infu		grams	100	mL
antibiotic (except vancomycin)	Outpt Infu			50	mL
antibiotic (except vancomycin)	Outpt Infu			100	mL
antibiotic (except vancomycin)	Outpt Infu			150	mL
antibiotic (except vancomycin)	Outpt Infu			250	mL
antibiotic (except vancomycin)	Outpt Infu			500	mL
vancomycin	Outpt Infu		mg		mL

Source: With permission from Fairview Health Services, Minneapolis, Minnesota.

Med. Max. Rate	Dose Rate Dosing Unit	Dose Rate LHL	Dose Rate LSL	Dose Rate USL	Dose Rate UHL
	mL/hr			205	
	mL/hr			25	
	mL/hr			210	
	mL/hr			160	
	mL/hr			960	
	mL/hr			225	
	mL/hr			75	
	mL/hr				400
	mL/hr			300	
	mL/hr			640	
	mL/hr			640	
	mL/hr			1000	
	mL/hr			1000	
	mL/hr			263	
	mL/hr			525	
	mL/hr			1000	
	mL/hr			320	
	mL/hr			640	
	mL/hr			215	
	mL/hr				
	mL/hr			50	
	mL/hr				
	mL/hr				
	mL/hr				460
	mL/hr				1000
	mL/hr				
	mL/hr				1000
	mEq/hr				10
	mEq/hr			20	40
	grams/hr				4
	grams/hr				4
	mL/hr		25	300	
	mL/hr		50	400	
	mL/hr		75	150	
	mL/hr		125	250	
	mL/hr		100	500	
	mg/hr			1700	2500

Source: With permission from Fairview Health Services, Minneapolis, Minnesota.

Table A-1. Continuous Dosing (cont'd)

Displayed Name	CCA Name	Med. Amount	Med. Unit	Diluent Amount	Diluent Unit
abatacept	Outpt Infu		mg	100	mL
calcium CHLORide	Outpt Infu		grams	100	mL
calcium GLUConate	Outpt Infu	1	grams	100	mL
ferric gluconate	Outpt Infu	125	mg	100	mL
ferric gluconate	Outpt Infu	250	mg	250	mL
immune globulin-sucrose out pat	Outpt Infu				mL
immune globulin-sucrose free op	Outpt Infu				mL
infliximab	Outpt Infu		mg	250	mL
iron dextran test dose	Outpt Infu	25	mg	50	mL
iron dextran	Outpt Infu		mg	500	mL
iron sucrose (Venofer)	Outpt Infu	200	mg	100	mL
iron sucrose (Venofer)	Outpt Infu	500	mg	250	mL
mannitol injection 20%	Outpt Infu	50	grams	250	mL
mannitol injection 20%	Outpt Infu	100	grams	500	mL
mannitol injection 25%	Outpt Infu	12.5	grams	50	mL
mannitol injection 25%	Outpt Infu		grams		mL
methylprednisolone	Outpt Infu		mg	100	mL
Other Drug	Outpt Infu		Select on Infuser		mL
pamidronate	Outpt Infu		mg	250	mL
pamidronate	Outpt Infu		mg	500	mL
pamidronate	Outpt Infu		mcg	1000	mL
prolastin	Outpt Infu		mg		mL
ranitidine intermittent	Outpt Infu	50	mg	50	mL
thymoglobulin	Outpt Infu	50	mg	115	mL
thymoglobulin	Outpt Infu	75	mg	173	mL
thymoglobulin	Outpt Infu	100	mg	283	mL
thymoglobulin-peripheral	Outpt Infu		mg	500	mL
zoledronic acid	Outpt Infu		mg	100	mL
IV fluid	adult bmt				mL
calcium GLUConate	adult bmt	1	grams	100	mL
cyclosporine	adult bmt		mg	100	mL
cyclosporine	adult bmt		mg	150	mL
cyclosporine	adult bmt		mg	250	mL
cyclosporine drip BMT	adult bmt	250	mg	250	mL
cyclosporine drip BMT	adult bmt	500	mg	250	mL

Source: With permission from Fairview Health Services, Minneapolis, Minnesota.

Med. Max. Rate	Dose Rate Dosing Unit	Dose Rate LHL	Dose Rate LSL	Dose Rate USL	Dose Rate UHL
	mL/hr			200	
	grams/hr				4
	grams/hr				4
	mL/hr				120
	mL/hr				150
	mL/kg/hr		0.5		2.5
	mL/kg/hr		0.5		4
	mL/hr		120	126	130
	mL/hr				200
	mL/hr		62.5	84	100
	mL/hr				120
	mL/hr			62.5	75
	mL/hr			1000	
	mL/hr			1000	
	mL/hr			1000	
	mL/hr			1000	
	mL/hr				400
	mL/hr				125
	mL/hr				250
	mL/hr				500
	mL/hr				1000
	mL/hr			300	420
	mL/hr			29	
	mL/hr			44	
	mL/hr			71	
	mL/hr			135	
	mL/hr				460
	mL/hr				1000
	grams/hr				4
	mL/hr				80
	mL/hr				105
	mL/hr				160
	mg/hr			16	20
	mg/hr			16	20

Source: With permission from Fairview Health Services, Minneapolis, Minnesota.

Table A-1. Continuous Dosing (cont'd)

Displayed Name	CCA Name	Med. Amount	Med. Unit	Diluent Amount	Diluent Unit
filgrastim	adult bmt	15	mcg	1	mL
foscarnet	adult bmt		mg		mL
ganciclovir	adult bmt		mg	100	mL
lipids 20%	adult bmt	50	grams	250	mL
lipids 20%	adult bmt	100	grams	500	mL
magnesium replacement	adult bmt		grams		mL
methylprednisolone	adult bmt		mg	100	mL
phytonadione (vitamin K)	adult bmt		mg	50	mL
potassium chloride	adult bmt	10	mEq	100	mL
potassium chloride	adult bmt	20	mEq	50	mL
potassium phosphate	adult bmt		mmol	500	mL
potassium phosphate	adult bmt		mmol	250	mL
sodium phosphate	adult bmt		mmol	250	mL
sodium phosphate	adult bmt		mmol	500	mL
TPN	adult bmt				mL
3% sodium chloride	adult bmt				mL
AMIODarone	adult bmt	500	mg	500	mL
AMIODarone	adult bmt	1500	mg	250	mL
antibiotic (except vancomycin)	adult bmt			50	mL
antibiotic (except vancomycin)	adult bmt			100	mL
antibiotic (except vancomycin)	adult bmt			150	mL
antibiotic (except vancomycin)	adult bmt			250	mL
antibiotic (except vancomycin)	adult bmt			500	mL
antithymocyte globulin horse	adult bmt		grams	250	mL
antithymocyte globulin horse	adult bmt		grams	500	mL
antithymocyte globulin horse	adult bmt		mg	150	mL
bumetanide ICU	adult bmt	25.	mg	100	mL
chemo infusion	adult bmt				mL
calcium CHLORide	adult bmt		grams	100	mL
chlorpromazine	adult bmt	25	mg	50	mL
chlorpromazine	adult bmt	50	mg	100	mL
cidofovir	adult bmt		mg	100	mL
dantrolene	adult bmt		mg		mL
desmopressin	adult bmt		mcg	50	mL
diltiazem	adult bmt	125	mg	125	mL
fentanyl	adult bmt	5	mg	100	mL

Source: With permission from Fairview Health Services, Minneapolis, Minnesota.

Med. Max. Rate	Dose Rate Dosing Unit	Dose Rate LHL	Dose Rate LSL	Dose Rate USL	Dose Rate UHL
	mL/hr			100	110
	mL/hr			500	
	mL/hr			160	
	mL/hr		1	25	62.5
	mL/hr		1	25	62.5
	grams/hr				2
	mL/hr				400
	mL/hr				100
	mEq/hr				10
	mEq/hr			20	40
	mL/hr			86	125
	mL/hr			65	86
	mL/hr			65	86
	mL/hr			86	125
	mL/hr			250	300
	mL/hr				100
	mg/min		0.4		2
	mg/min		0.4		2
	mL/hr		25	300	
	mL/hr		50	400	
	mL/hr		75	150	
	mL/hr		125	250	
	mL/hr		100	500	
	mL/hr			80	
	mL/hr			155	
	mL/hr			52	
	mg/hr		0.5		4
	mL/hr				
	grams/hr				4
	mL/hr			100	
	mL/hr			100	
	mL/hr			115	130
	mg/hr			500	
	mL/hr			200	
	mg/hr		1	15	20
	mcg/hr				

Source: With permission from Fairview Health Services, Minneapolis, Minnesota.

Table A-1. Continuous Dosing (cont'd)

Displayed Name	CCA Name	Med. Amount	Med. Unit	Diluent Amount	Diluent Unit
furosemide	adult bmt	100	mg	100	mL
HEParin	adult bmt	25000	units	250	mL
HYDROmorphone	adult bmt		mg		mL
immune globulin-sucrose	adult bmt				mL
immune globulin-sucrose free	adult bmt				mL
ketamine	adult bmt		mg		mL
leucovorin	adult bmt	10	mg	1	mL
levetiracetam	adult bmt			100	mL
lorazepam	adult bmt	50	mg	50	mL
metoclopramide	adult bmt		mg	50	mL
midazolam	adult bmt	50	mg	50	mL
morphine	adult bmt		mg		mL
mycophenolate 500 mg dose	adult bmt	500	mg		mL
mycophenolate 1000 mg dose	adult bmt	1000	mg		mL
mycophenolate 1500 mg dose	adult bmt	1500	mg		mL
octreotide	adult bmt	1250	mcg	250	mL
ondansetron drip	adult bmt	50	mg	50	mL
Other Drug	adult bmt		Select on Infuser		mL
PANtoprazole	adult bmt	80	mg	100	mL
premedication	adult bmt		mg	50	mL
rituximab	adult bmt	1	mg	1	mL
sodium bicarbonate	adult bmt		mEq		mL
tacrolimus	adult bmt	5	mg	250	mL
thymoglobulin-BMT	adult bmt		mg	100	mL
thymoglobulin-BMT	adult bmt		mg	150	mL
thymoglobulin-BMT	adult bmt		mg	250	mL
thymoglobulin-BMT	adult bmt		mg	500	mL
vancomycin	adult bmt		mg		mL
zoledronic acid	adult bmt		mg	100	mL
Chemo over 30 min in ~50 mL	adult bmt			50	mL
Chemo over 30 min in ~100 mL	adult bmt			100	mL
Chemo over 30 min ~150 mL	adult bmt			150	mL
Chemo over 30 min in ~250 mL	adult bmt			250	mL
Chemo over 30 min in ~500 mL	adult bmt			500	mL
chemo over 1 hour ~ 100 mL	adult bmt			100	mL

Source: With permission from Fairview Health Services, Minneapolis, Minnesota.

Med. Max. Rate	Dose Rate Dosing Unit	Dose Rate LHL	Dose Rate LSL	Dose Rate USL	Dose Rate UHL
	mg/hr			30	60
	units/hr	50	200	2000	2500
	mg/hr				
	mL/kg/hr		0.5		2.5
	mL/kg/hr		0.5		4
	mg/hr				20
	mg/min				160
	mL/hr			400	
	mg/hr		0.2	20	30
	mL/hr				200
	mg/hr		0.2	20	30
	mg/hr				
	mg/hr				250
	mg/hr				500
	mg/hr				750
	mcg/hr			150	250
	mg/hr				5
	mg/hr		7.9		8
	mL/hr				250
	mL/hr				400
	mEq/hr			50	
	mcg/hr	5	10	120	200
	mL/hr			29	
	mL/hr			44	
	mL/hr			71	
	mL/hr			135	
	mg/hr			1700	2500
	mL/hr				460
	mL/hr			120	150
	mL/hr				320
	mL/hr				420
	mL/hr			520	550
	mL/hr			1000	
	mL/hr				160

Source: With permission from Fairview Health Services, Minneapolis, Minnesota.

Table A-1. Continuous Dosing (cont'd)

Displayed Name	CCA Name	Med. Amount	Med. Unit	Diluent Amount	Diluent Unit
chemo over 1 hour ~ 150 mL	adult bmt			150	mL
chemo over 1 hour ~ 250 mL	adult bmt			250	mL
Chemo over 1 hr in ~500 mL	adult bmt			500	mL
Chemo over 2 hr in ~100 mL	adult bmt			100	mL
Chemo over 2 hr in ~ 150 mL	adult bmt			150	mL
Chemo over 2 hr in ~ 250 mL	adult bmt			250	mL
Chemo over 2 hr in ~ 500 mL	adult bmt			500	mL
Chemo over 3 hr in ~ 250 mL	adult bmt			250	mL
Chemo over 3 hr in ~ 500 mL	adult bmt			500	mL
Chemo over 24 hr in ~1000 mL	adult bmt			1000	mL
IV fluid	intermed				mL
blood products	intermed				mL
antibiotic (except vancomycin)	intermed			50	mL
antibiotic (except vancomycin)	intermed			100	mL
antibiotic (except vancomycin)	intermed			150	mL
antibiotic (except vancomycin)	intermed			250	mL
antibiotic (except vancomycin)	intermed			500	mL
AMIODarone	intermed	500	mg	500	mL
AMIODarone	intermed	1500	mg	250	mL
diltiazem	intermed	125	mg	125	mL
HEParin	intermed	25000	units	250	mL
nitroGLYCERIN-IMC	intermed	50	mg	250	mL
nitroGLYCERIN-IMC	intermed	200	mg	250	mL
milrinone	intermed	20	mg	100	mL
furosemide	intermed	100	mg	100	mL
DOBUTamine-IMC	intermed	500	mg	250	mL
DOBUTamine-IMC	intermed	1000	mg	250	mL
DOPamine-IMC	intermed	400	mg	250	mL
DOPamine-IMC	intermed	800	mg	250	mL
esmolol	intermed	2000	mg	100	mL
potassium chloride	intermed	10	mEq	100	mL
potassium chloride	intermed	20	mEq	50	mL
TPN	intermed				mL
lipids 20%	intermed	50	grams	250	mL
lipids 20%	intermed	100	grams	500	mL
magnesium replacement	intermed		grams		mL
thymoglobulin	intermed	50	mg	115	mL

Source: With permission from Fairview Health Services, Minneapolis, Minnesota.

Med. Max. Rate	Dose Rate Dosing Unit	Dose Rate LHL	Dose Rate LSL	Dose Rate USL	Dose Rate UHL
	mL/hr				210
499	mL/hr			270	325
	mL/hr				610
	mL/hr				80
	mL/hr				110
	mL/hr				160
	mL/hr				310
	mL/hr			90	150
	mL/hr			175	240
	mL/hr				50
	mL/hr				1000
	mL/hr				1000
	mL/hr		25	300	
	mL/hr		50	400	
	mL/hr		75	150	
	mL/hr		125	250	
	mL/hr		100	500	
	mg/min		0.4		2
	mg/min		0.4		2
	mg/hr		1	15	20
	units/hr	50	200	2000	2500
	mcg/kg/min			2	
	mcg/kg/min			2	
	mcg/kg/min		0.1		1
	mg/hr			30	60
	mcg/kg/min			11	15
	mcg/kg/min			11	15
	mcg/kg/min			6	8
	mcg/kg/min			6	8
	mcg/kg/min			300	350
	mEq/hr				10
	mEq/hr			20	40
	mL/hr			250	300
	mL/hr		1	25	62.5
	mL/hr		1	25	62.5
	grams/hr				2
	mL/hr			29	

Source: With permission from Fairview Health Services, Minneapolis, Minnesota.

Table A-1. Continuous Dosing (cont'd)

Displayed Name	CCA Name	Med. Amount	Med. Unit	Diluent Amount	Diluent Unit
thymoglobulin	intermed	75	mg	173	mL
thymoglobulin	intermed	100	mg	283	mL
thymoglobulin-peripheral	intermed		mg	500	mL
immune globulin-sucrose	intermed				mL
immune globulin-sucrose free	intermed				mL
3% sodium chloride	intermed				mL
abciximab 80 kg or more	intermed	9	mg	250	mL
abciximab less than 80 kg	intermed	9	mg	250	mL
acetylcysteine-renal	intermed	600	mg	100	mL
acetylcysteine-renal	intermed	1200	mg	100	mL
alemtuzumab	intermed		mg	100	mL
alteplase PE	intermed	100	mg	100	mL
alteplase stroke	intermed		mg		mL
argatroban-cath lab	intermed	250	mg	250	mL
argatroban non-cath lab	intermed	250	mg	250	mL
basiliximab	intermed		mg	50	mL
BEVACizumab over 30 min	intermed		mg	100	mL
BEVACizumab over 60 min	intermed		mg	100	mL
BEVACizumab over 90 min	intermed		mg	100	mL
bumetanide	intermed	25	mg	100	mL
calcium CHLORide	intermed		grams	100	mL
calcium GLUConate	intermed	1	grams	100	mL
chlorpromazine	intermed	25	mg	50	mL
chlorpromazine	intermed	50	mg	100	mL
conivaptan	intermed	20	mg	250	mL
cyclosporine drip-solid organ	intermed	250	mg	250	mL
cyclosporine drip-solid organ	intermed	500	mg	250	mL
daclizumab	intermed		mg	50	mL
deferoxamine	intermed		mg	250	mL
desmopressin	intermed		mcg	50	mL
eptifibatide	intermed	200	mg	100	mL
ferric gluconate	intermed	125	mg	100	mL
ferric gluconate	intermed	250	mg	250	mL
foscarnet	intermed		mg		mL
fosphenytoin	intermed		mg		mL
ganciclovir	intermed		mg	100	mL
infliximab	intermed		mg	250	mL

Source: With permission from Fairview Health Services, Minneapolis, Minnesota.

Med. Max. Rate	Dose Rate Dosing Unit	Dose Rate LHL	Dose Rate LSL	Dose Rate USL	Dose Rate UHL
	mL/hr			44	
	mL/hr			71	
	mL/hr			135	
	mL/kg/hr		0.5		2.5
	mL/kg/hr		0.5		4
	mL/hr			100	
	mcg/min		5		10
	mcg/kg/min				0.125
	mL/hr			400	
	mL/hr			400	
	mL/hr			80	
	mg/hr		50	50	100
	mg/hr				81
	mcg/kg/min			30	40
	mcg/kg/min			5	10
	mL/hr		50		150
	mL/hr			320	
	mL/hr			160	
	mL/hr			107	
	mg/hr		0.5		2
	grams/hr				4
	grams/hr				4
	mL/hr			100	
	mL/hr			100	
	mg/hr	0.8			1.7
	mg/hr			5	9.9
	mg/hr			5	9.9
	mL/hr			210	
	mg/hr			1500	
	mL/hr			200	
	mcg/kg/min				2
	mL/hr				120
	mL/hr				150
	mL/hr			500	
	mg/min				150
	mL/hr			160	
	mL/hr		120	126	130

Source: With permission from Fairview Health Services, Minneapolis, Minnesota.

Table A-1. Continuous Dosing (cont'd)

Displayed Name	CCA Name	Med. Amount	Med. Unit	Diluent Amount	Diluent Unit
iron dextran	intermed		mg	500	mL
iron dextran test dose	intermed	25	mg	50	mL
iron sucrose (Venofer)	intermed	200	mg	100	mL
iron sucrose (Venofer)	intermed	500	mg	250	mL
isoproterenol-mcg/kg/min dosing	intermed	1	mg	50	mL
lepirudin	intermed	100	mg	250	mL
levetiracetam	intermed			100	mL
mannitol injection 20%	intermed	50	grams	250	mL
mannitol injection 20%	intermed	100	grams	500	mL
mannitol injection 25%	intermed	12.5	grams	50	mL
mannitol injection 25%	intermed		grams		mL
methylprednisolone	intermed		mg	100	mL
mycophenolate 500 mg dose	intermed	500	mg		mL
mycophenolate 1000 mg dose	intermed	1000	mg		mL
mycophenolate 1500 mg dose	intermed	1500	mg		mL
naloxone	intermed	4	mg	100	mL
octreotide	intermed	1250	mcg	250	mL
ondansetron drip	intermed	50	mg	50	mL
Other Drug	intermed		Select on Infuser		mL
PANtoprazole	intermed	80	mg	100	mL
phytonadione (vitamin K)	intermed		mg	50	mL
potassium phosphate	intermed		mmol	250	mL
potassium phosphate	intermed		mmol	500	mL
rituximab	intermed	1	mg	1	mL
sodium bicarbonate	intermed		mEq		mL
sodium phosphate	intermed		mmol	250	mL
sodium phosphate	intermed		mmol	500	mL
tacrolimus	intermed	5	mg	250	mL
tenecteplase	intermed	5	mg	500	mL
valproate	intermed		mg	100	mL
vancomycin	intermed		mg		mL

Source: With permission from Fairview Health Services, Minneapolis, Minnesota.

Med. Max. Rate	Dose Rate Dosing Unit	Dose Rate LHL	Dose Rate LSL	Dose Rate USL	Dose Rate UHL
	mL/hr		62.5	84	100
	mL/hr				200
	mL/hr				120
	mL/hr			62.5	75
	mcg/kg/min		0.01	0.3	
	mg/kg/hr		0.02	0.21	
	mL/hr			400	
	mL/hr			1000	
	mL/hr			1000	
	mL/hr			1000	
	mL/hr			1000	
	mL/hr				400
	mg/hr				250
	mg/hr				500
	mg/hr				750
	mg/hr		0.05	1	
	mcg/hr			150	250
	mg/hr				5
	mg/hr		7.9		8
	mL/hr				100
	mL/hr			65	86
	mL/hr			86	125
	mL/hr				400
	mEq/hr			50	
	mL/hr			65	86
	mL/hr			86	125
	mcg/hr	5	10	120	200
	mg/hr	0.05	0.1	1	1.2
	mL/hr			100	
	mg/hr			1700	2500

Source: With permission from Fairview Health Services, Minneapolis, Minnesota.

Table A-2. Bolus Dosing

Displayed Name	CCA Name	Med. Amount	Med. Unit	Diluent Amount	Diluent Unit	Bolus Enabled
aminocaproic acid	ICU	5	grams	100	mL	
AMIODarone	ICU	500	mg	500	mL	x
AMIODarone	ICU	1500	mg	250	mL	x
cisatracurium	ICU	200	mg	100	mL	x
dexmedetomidine	ICU	200	mcg	50	mL	x
dexmedetomidine	ICU	400	mcg	100	mL	x
DOBUTamine	ICU	500	mg	250	mL	
DOBUTamine	ICU	1000	mg	250	mL	
DOPamine	ICU	400	mg	250	mL	
DOPamine	ICU	800	mg	250	mL	
EPInephrine	ICU	5	mg	250	mL	
EPInephrine	ICU	16	mg	250	mL	
EPInephrine-mcg/ kg/min dosing	ICU	5	mg	250	mL	
EPInephrine-mcg/ kg/min dosing	ICU	16	mg	250	mL	
esmolol	ICU	2000	mg	100	mL	x
HEParin	ICU	25000	units	250	mL	x
isoproterenol	ICU	1	mg	50	mL	
isoproterenol-mcg/ kg/min dosing	ICU	1	mg	50	mL	
lidocaine	ICU	2	grams	250	mL	
milrinone	ICU	20	mg	100	mL	x
NICARdipine	ICU	25	mg	250	mL	
NICARdipine	ICU	100	mg	250	mL	
nitroGLYCERIN	ICU	50	mg	250	mL	
nitroGLYCERIN	ICU	200	mg	250	mL	
nitroGLYCERIN-mcg/kg/min dosing	ICU	50	mg	250	mL	
nitroGLYCERIN-mcg/kg/min dosing	ICU	200	mg	250	mL	
nitroPRUSSide	ICU	100	mg	250	mL	
nitroPRUSSide	ICU	400	mg	250	mL	
NOREPInephrine	ICU	8	mg	250	mL	
NOREPInephrine	ICU	16	mg	250	mL	
NOREPInephrine-mcg/kg/min dosing	ICU	8	mg	250	mL	

Source: With permission from Fairview Health Services, Minneapolis, Minnesota.

Bolus Dose Amt. Unit	Bolus Dose Amt. LHL	Bolus Dose Amt. LSL	Bolus Dose Amt. USL	Bolus Dose Amt. UHL	Bolus Time LHL	Bolus Time LSL	Bolus Time USL	Bolus Time UHL	Bolus Dose Rate Dosing Unit
mg				150	0:10		0:30		
mg				150	0:10		0:30		
mg			30						
mcg			150		0:10				
mcg			150		0:10				
mg			60						
units			6000	10000			0:06		
mg			5						

Source: With permission from Fairview Health Services, Minneapolis, Minnesota.

Table A-2. Bolus Dosing (cont'd)

Displayed Name	CCA Name	Med. Amount	Med. Unit	Diluent Amount	Diluent Unit	Bolus Enabled
NOREPInephrine-mcg/kg/min dosing	ICU	16	mg	250	mL	
phenylephrine	ICU	50	mg	250	mL	
phenylephrine-mcg/kg/min dosing	ICU	50	mg	250	mL	
phenylephrine-mcg/kg/min dosing	ICU	200	mg	250	mL	
propofol	ICU	1000	mg	100	mL	x
vasopressin	ICU	100	units	100	mL	
vecuronium	ICU	50	mg	50	mL	x
IV fluid	ICU				mL	x
23.4% Sodium Chloride	ICU			30	mL	
3% sodium chloride	ICU				mL	
abciximab less than 80 kg	ICU	9	mg	250	mL	x
abciximab 80 kg or more	ICU	9	mg	250	mL	x
acetylcysteine Step 1	ICU		grams	200	mL	
acetylcysteine Step 2	ICU		grams	500	mL	
acetylcysteine Step 3	ICU		grams	1000	mL	
acetylcysteine-renal	ICU	600	mg	100	mL	
acetylcysteine-renal	ICU	1200	mg	100	mL	
alemtuzumab	ICU		mg	100	mL	
alprostadil	ICU	1	mg	100	mL	
alteplase PE	ICU	100	mg	100	mL	x
alteplase-rad	ICU	1	mg	100	mL	
alteplase stroke	ICU		mg		mL	x
antibiotic (except vancomycin)	ICU			50	mL	
antibiotic (except vancomycin)	ICU			100	mL	
antibiotic (except vancomycin)	ICU			150	mL	
antibiotic (except vancomycin)	ICU			250	mL	
antibiotic (except vancomycin)	ICU			500	mL	

Source: With permission from Fairview Health Services, Minneapolis, Minnesota.

Bolus Dose Amt. Unit	Bolus Dose Amt. LHL	Bolus Dose Amt. LSL	Bolus Dose Amt. USL	Bolus Dose Amt. UHL	Bolus Time LHL	Bolus Time LSL	Bolus Time USL	Bolus Time UHL	Bolus Dose Rate Dosing Unit
mg			30						
mg			10						
mL				1000					
mg				20					
mg			50						
mg			10		1:00				
mg				9				0:01	

Source: With permission from Fairview Health Services, Minneapolis, Minnesota.

Table A-2. Bolus Dosing (cont'd)

Displayed Name	CCA Name	Med. Amount	Med. Unit	Diluent Amount	Diluent Unit	Bolus Enabled
antithymocyte globu-lin horse	ICU		mg	50	mL	
antithymocyte globu-lin horse	ICU		mg	100	mL	
antithymocyte globu-lin horse	ICU		mg	150	mL	
antithymocyte globu-lin horse	ICU		grams	250	mL	
antithymocyte globu-lin horse	ICU		grams	500	mL	
argatroban non-cath lab	ICU	250	mg	250	mL	
argatroban-cath lab	ICU	250	mg	250	mL	
basiliximab	ICU		mg	50	mL	
BEVACizumab over 30 min	ICU		mg	100	mL	
BEVACizumab over 60 min	ICU		mg	100	mL	
BEVACizumab over 90 min	ICU		mg	100	mL	
bivalirudin non-cath lab	ICU	250	mg	50	mL	
bivalirudin-cath lab	ICU	250	mg	50	mL	x
bumetanide ICU	ICU	25	mg	100	mL	x
calcium CHLORide	ICU		grams	100	mL	
calcium GLUConate	ICU	1	grams	100	mL	
chlorpromazine	ICU	25	mg	50	mL	
chlorpromazine	ICU	50	mg	100	mL	
cidofovir	ICU		mg	100	mL	
clevidipine	ICU	25	mg	50	mL	
conivaptan	ICU	20	mg	250	mL	x
cyclosporine	ICU		mg	100	mL	
cyclosporine	ICU		mg	150	mL	
cyclosporine	ICU		mg	250	mL	
cyclosporine drip BMT	ICU	250	mg	250	mL	
cyclosporine drip BMT	ICU	500	mg	250	mL	
cyclosporine drip-solid organ	ICU	250	mg	250	mL	

Source: With permission from Fairview Health Services, Minneapolis, Minnesota.

Bolus Dose Amt. Unit	Bolus Dose Amt. LHL	Bolus Dose Amt. LSL	Bolus Dose Amt. USL	Bolus Dose Amt. UHL	Bolus Time LHL	Bolus Time LSL	Bolus Time USL	Bolus Time UHL	Bolus Dose Rate Dosing Unit
mg			113						
mg				2					
mg				20	0:30				

Source: With permission from Fairview Health Services, Minneapolis, Minnesota.

Table A-2. Bolus Dosing (cont'd)

Displayed Name	CCA Name	Med. Amount	Med. Unit	Diluent Amount	Diluent Unit	Bolus Enabled
cyclosporine drip-solid organ	ICU	500	mg	250	mL	
daclizumab	ICU		mg	50	mL	
dantrolene	ICU		mg		mL	
deferoxamine	ICU		mg	250	mL	
desmopressin	ICU		mcg	50	mL	
echo-DOBUTamine	ICU	500	mg	250	mL	
diltiazem	ICU	125	mg	125	mL	x
drotrecogin alfa (Xigris)	ICU	10	mg	100	mL	
drotrecogin alfa (Xigris)	ICU	20	mg	200	mL	
eptifibatide	ICU	200	mg	100	mL	x
fentanyl	ICU	5	mg	100	mL	x
ferric gluconate	ICU	125	mg	100	mL	
ferric gluconate	ICU	250	mg	250	mL	
foscarnet	ICU		mg		mL	
fosphenytoin	ICU		mg		mL	
furosemide	ICU	100	mg	100	mL	x
ganciclovir	ICU		mg	100	mL	
HYDROmorphone	ICU		mg		mL	x
immune globulin-sucrose	ICU				mL	
immune globulin-sucrose free	ICU				mL	
infliximab	ICU		mg	250	mL	
insulin-ICU	ICU	50	units	50	mL	x
iron dextran test dose	ICU	25	mg	50	mL	
iron dextran	ICU		mg	500	mL	
iron sucrose (Venofer)	ICU	200	mg	100	mL	
iron sucrose (Venofer)	ICU	500	mg	250	mL	
ketamine	ICU		mg		mL	x
labetalol	ICU	250	mg	50	mL	x
lepirudin	ICU	100	mg	250	mL	x
leucovorin	ICU	10	mg	1	mL	

Source: With permission from Fairview Health Services, Minneapolis, Minnesota.

Bolus Dose Amt. Unit	Bolus Dose Amt. LHL	Bolus Dose Amt. LSL	Bolus Dose Amt. USL	Bolus Dose Amt. UHL	Bolus Time LHL	Bolus Time LSL	Bolus Time USL	Bolus Time UHL	Bolus Dose Rate Dosing Unit
mg			35	60					
mg				22.6					
mcg									
mg			80						
mg									
units	0.5		10	20					
mg			10		0:03				
mg			80						
mg			44						

Source: With permission from Fairview Health Services, Minneapolis, Minnesota.

Table A-2. Bolus Dosing (cont'd)

Displayed Name	CCA Name	Med. Amount	Med. Unit	Diluent Amount	Diluent Unit	Bolus Enabled
levetiracetam	ICU			100	mL	
lipids 20%	ICU	50	grams	250	mL	
lipids anesthetic overdose	ICU	50	grams	250	mL	x
lorazepam	ICU	50	mg	50	mL	x
lorazepam	ICU	100	mg	100	mL	x
magnesium replacement	ICU		grams		mL	
methylprednisolone	ICU		mg	100	mL	
methylpred INF spinal cord	ICU		mg	500	mL	
methylpred bolus spinal cord	ICU		mg	100	mL	
metoclopramide	ICU		mg	50	mL	
midazolam	ICU	100	mg	100	mL	x
morphine	ICU		mg		mL	x
mycophenolate 500 mg dose	ICU	500	mg		mL	
mycophenolate 1000 mg dose	ICU	1000	mg		mL	
mycophenolate 1500 mg dose	ICU	1500	mg		mL	
naloxone	ICU	4	mg	100	mL	x
nesiritide	ICU	1.5	mg	250	mL	x
octreotide	ICU	1250	mcg	250	mL	
ondansetron drip	ICU	50	mg	50	mL	
Other Drug	ICU		Select on Infuser		mL	x
PANtoprazole	ICU	80	mg	100	mL	
PenTobarbital	ICU	2000	mg	250	mL	x
PHenobarbital	ICU	2000	mg	250	mL	x
phenytoin	ICU		mg		mL	
phytonadione (vitamin K)	ICU		mg	50	mL	
potassium chloride	ICU	10	mEq	100	mL	
potassium chloride	ICU	20	mEq	50	mL	
potassium phosphate	ICU		mmol	250	mL	

Source: With permission from Fairview Health Services, Minneapolis, Minnesota.

Bolus Dose Amt. Unit	Bolus Dose Amt. LHL	Bolus Dose Amt. LSL	Bolus Dose Amt. USL	Bolus Dose Amt. UHL	Bolus Time LHL	Bolus Time LSL	Bolus Time USL	Bolus Time UHL	Bolus Dose Rate Dosing Unit
mL/kg			1.5						
mg			4			0:02	0:05		
mg			4			0:02	0:05		
mg			4			0:02	0:05		
mg									
mg			2						
mcg			360			0:10			
mg			500		0:30				
mg			2000		0:30				

Source: With permission from Fairview Health Services, Minneapolis, Minnesota.

Table A-2. Bolus Dosing (cont'd)

Displayed Name	CCA Name	Med. Amount	Med. Unit	Diluent Amount	Diluent Unit	Bolus Enabled
potassium phosphate	ICU		mmol	500	mL	
procainamide	ICU	2	grams	250	mL	x
rituximab	ICU	1	mg	1	mL	
rocuronium	ICU	500	mg	250	mL	x
sodium bicarbonate	ICU		mEq		mL	
sodium phosphate	ICU		mmol	250	mL	
sodium phosphate	ICU		mmol	500	mL	
tacrolimus	ICU	5	mg	250	mL	
tenecteplase	ICU	5	mg	500	mL	
thymoglobulin	ICU	50	mg	115	mL	
thymoglobulin	ICU	75	mg	173	mL	
thymoglobulin	ICU	100	mg	283	mL	
thymoglobulin-peripheral	ICU		mg	500	mL	
TPN	ICU				mL	
valproate	ICU		mg	100	mL	
vancomycin	ICU		mg		mL	
zoledronic acid	ICU		mg	100	mL	
IV fluid	Med-Surg				mL	x
blood products	Med-Surg				mL	
antibiotic (except vancomycin)	Med-Surg			50	mL	
antibiotic (except vancomycin)	Med-Surg			100	mL	
antibiotic (except vancomycin)	Med-Surg			150	mL	
antibiotic (except vancomycin)	Med-Surg			250	mL	
antibiotic (except vancomycin)	Med-Surg			500	mL	
vancomycin	Med-Surg		mg		mL	
potassium chloride	Med-Surg	10	mEq	100	mL	
potassium chloride	Med-Surg	20	mEq	50	mL	

Source: With permission from Fairview Health Services, Minneapolis, Minnesota.

Bolus Dose Amt. Unit	Bolus Dose Amt. LHL	Bolus Dose Amt. LSL	Bolus Dose Amt. USL	Bolus Dose Amt. UHL	Bolus Time LHL	Bolus Time LSL	Bolus Time USL	Bolus Time UHL	Bolus Dose Rate Dosing Unit
mg			1700			0:45			
mg/kg			0.6						
mL				1000					

Source: With permission from Fairview Health Services, Minneapolis, Minnesota.

Table A-2. Bolus Dosing (cont'd)

Displayed Name	CCA Name	Med. Amount	Med. Unit	Diluent Amount	Diluent Unit	Bolus Enabled
magnesium replacement	Med-Surg		grams		mL	
TPN	Med-Surg				mL	
lipids 20%	Med-Surg	50	grams	250	mL	
lipids 20%	Med-Surg	100	grams	500	mL	
HEParin	Med-Surg	25000	units	250	mL	x
acetylcysteine-renal	Med-Surg	600	mg	100	mL	
acetylcysteine-renal	Med-Surg	1200	mg	100	mL	
alemtuzumab	Med-Surg		mg	100	mL	
alteplase stroke	Med-Surg		mg		mL	x
alteplase PE	Med-Surg	100	mg	100	mL	x
alteplase-rad	Med-Surg	12.5	mg	50	mL	
AMIODarone	Med-Surg	500	mg	500	mL	x
argatroban non-cath lab	Med-Surg	250	mg	250	mL	
basiliximab	Med-Surg		mg	50	mL	
BEVACizumab over 30 min	Med-Surg		mg	100	mL	
BEVACizumab over 60 min	Med-Surg		mg	100	mL	
BEVACizumab over 90 min	Med-Surg		mg	100	mL	
bumetanide	Med-Surg	25	mg	100	mL	x
calcium CHLORide	Med-Surg		grams	100	mL	
calcium GLUConate	Med-Surg	1	grams	100	mL	
chlorpromazine	Med-Surg	25	mg	50	mL	

Source: With permission from Fairview Health Services, Minneapolis, Minnesota.

Bolus Dose Amt. Unit	Bolus Dose Amt. LHL	Bolus Dose Amt. LSL	Bolus Dose Amt. USL	Bolus Dose Amt. UHL	Bolus Time LHL	Bolus Time LSL	Bolus Time USL	Bolus Time UHL	Bolus Dose Rate Dosing Unit
units			6000	10000			0:06		
mg			9					0:01	
mg			10		1:00				
mg				150	0:10		0:30		
mg			2						

Source: With permission from Fairview Health Services, Minneapolis, Minnesota.

Table A-2. Bolus Dosing (cont'd)

Displayed Name	CCA Name	Med. Amount	Med. Unit	Diluent Amount	Diluent Unit	Bolus Enabled
chlorpromazine	Med-Surg	50	mg	100	mL	
conivaptan	Med-Surg	20	mg	250	mL	x
cyclosporine drip-solid organ	Med-Surg	250	mg	250	mL	
cyclosporine drip-solid organ	Med-Surg	500	mg	250	mL	
daclizumab	Med-Surg		mg	50	mL	
deferoxamine	Med-Surg		mg	250	mL	
desmopressin	Med-Surg		mcg	50	mL	
diltiazem	Med-Surg	125	mg	125	mL	x
ferric gluconate	Med-Surg	125	mg	100	mL	
ferric gluconate	Med-Surg	250	mg	250	mL	
foscarnet	Med-Surg		mg		mL	
fosphenytoin	Med-Surg		mg		mL	
furosemide	Med-Surg	100	mg	100	mL	x
ganciclovir	Med-Surg		mg	100	mL	
immune globulin-sucrose	Med-Surg				mL	
immune globulin-sucrose free	Med-Surg				mL	
infliximab	Med-Surg		mg	250	mL	
insulin	Med-Surg	50	units	50	mL	x
iron dextran test dose	Med-Surg	25	mg	50	mL	
iron dextran	Med-Surg		mg	500	mL	
iron sucrose (Venofer)	Med-Surg	200	mg	100	mL	

Source: With permission from Fairview Health Services, Minneapolis, Minnesota.

Bolus Dose Amt. Unit	Bolus Dose Amt. LHL	Bolus Dose Amt. LSL	Bolus Dose Amt. USL	Bolus Dose Amt. UHL	Bolus Time LHL	Bolus Time LSL	Bolus Time USL	Bolus Time UHL	Bolus Dose Rate Dosing Unit
mg				20	0:30				
mg			35	60					
mg		80							
units	0.5			10					

Source: With permission from Fairview Health Services, Minneapolis, Minnesota.

Table A-2. Bolus Dosing (cont'd)

Displayed Name	CCA Name	Med. Amount	Med. Unit	Diluent Amount	Diluent Unit	Bolus Enabled
iron sucrose (Venofer)	Med-Surg	500	mg	250	mL	
lepirudin	Med-Surg	100	mg	250	mL	x
levetiracetam	Med-Surg			100	mL	
mannitol injection 20%	Med-Surg	50	grams	250	mL	
mannitol injection 20%	Med-Surg	100	grams	500	mL	
mannitol injection 25%	Med-Surg	12.5	grams	50	mL	
mannitol injection 25%	Med-Surg		grams		mL	
metoclopramide	Med-Surg		mg	50	mL	
methylprednisolone	Med-Surg		mg	100	mL	
mycophenolate 500 mg dose	Med-Surg	500	mg		mL	
mycophenolate 1000 mg dose	Med-Surg	1000	mg		mL	
mycophenolate 1500 mg dose	Med-Surg	1500	mg		mL	
naloxone	Med-Surg	4	mg	100	mL	x
octreotide	Med-Surg	1250	mcg	250	mL	
ondansetron drip	Med-Surg	50	mg	50	mL	
Other Drug	Med-Surg		Select on Infuser		mL	x
PANtoprazole	Med-Surg	80	mg	100	mL	
phytonadione (vitamin K)	Med-Surg		mg	50	mL	
potassium phosphate	Med-Surg		mmol	250	mL	
potassium phosphate	Med-Surg		mmol	500	mL	
rituximab	Med-Surg	1	mg	1	mL	

Source: With permission from Fairview Health Services, Minneapolis, Minnesota.

Bolus Dose Amt. Unit	Bolus Dose Amt. LHL	Bolus Dose Amt. LSL	Bolus Dose Amt. USL	Bolus Dose Amt. UHL	Bolus Time LHL	Bolus Time LSL	Bolus Time USL	Bolus Time UHL	Bolus Dose Rate Dosing Unit
mg				44					
mg		2							

Table A-2. Bolus Dosing (cont'd)

Displayed Name	CCA Name	Med. Amount	Med. Unit	Diluent Amount	Diluent Unit	Bolus Enabled
sodium bicarbonate	Med-Surg		mEq		mL	
1.5% sodium chloride	Med-Surg			1000	mL	
3% sodium chloride	Med-Surg				mL	
sodium phosphate	Med-Surg		mmol	250	mL	
sodium phosphate	Med-Surg		mmol	500	mL	
tacrolimus	Med-Surg	5	mg	250	mL	
thymoglobulin	Med-Surg	50	mg	115	mL	
thymoglobulin	Med-Surg	75	mg	173	mL	
thymoglobulin	Med-Surg	100	mg	283	mL	
thymoglobulin-pe-ripheral	Med-Surg		mg	500	mL	
valproate	Med-Surg		mg	100	mL	
IV fluid	OB				mL	x
oxytocin-labor	OB	20	units	1000	mL	
oxytocin-postpartum	OB	20	units	1000	mL	
oxytocin-postpartum	OB	40	units	1000	mL	
magnesium sulfate infusion	OB	20	grams	500	mL	x
magnesium seizure	OB	2	grams	50	mL	
magnesium seizure	OB	4	grams	50	mL	
antibiotic (except vancomycin)	OB			50	mL	
antibiotic (except vancomycin)	OB			100	mL	
antibiotic (except vancomycin)	OB			150	mL	
antibiotic (except vancomycin)	OB			250	mL	
antibiotic (except vancomycin)	OB			500	mL	
vancomycin	OB		mg		mL	

Source: With permission from Fairview Health Services, Minneapolis, Minnesota.

Bolus Dose Amt. Unit	Bolus Dose Amt. LHL	Bolus Dose Amt. LSL	Bolus Dose Amt. USL	Bolus Dose Amt. UHL	Bolus Time LHL	Bolus Time LSL	Bolus Time USL	Bolus Time UHL	Bolus Dose Rate Dosing Unit
mL			1000						
grams			6					0:30	grams/hr

Table A-2. Bolus Dosing (cont'd)

Displayed Name	CCA Name	Med. Amount	Med. Unit	Diluent Amount	Diluent Unit	Bolus Enabled
blood products	OB				mL	
HEParin	OB	25000	units	250	mL	x
insulin-OB	OB	50	units	50	mL	x
TPN	OB				mL	
lipids 20%	OB	50	grams	250	mL	
lipids 20%	OB	100	grams	500	mL	
potassium chloride	OB	10	mEq	100	mL	
hetastarch (Hespan)	OB			500	mL	
Other Drug	OB		Select on Infuser		mL	x
fosphenytoin	OB		mg		mL	
zidovudine	OB		mg		mL	x
IV fluid	Oncology				mL	x
premedication	Oncology		mg	50	mL	
premedication	Oncology		mg	100	mL	
premedication	Oncology		mg	150	mL	
ALDESleukin	Oncology		Million Units	50	mL	
alemtuzumab	Oncology		mg	100	mL	
amifostine	Oncology		mg	50	mL	
antithymocyte globulin horse	Oncology		mg	50	mL	
antithymocyte globulin horse	Oncology		mg	100	mL	
antithymocyte globulin horse	Oncology		mg	150	mL	
antithymocyte globulin horse	Oncology		grams	250	mL	
antithymocyte globulin horse	Oncology		grams	500	mL	
arsenic trioxide	Oncology		mg	250	mL	

Source: With permission from Fairview Health Services, Minneapolis, Minnesota.

Bolus Dose Amt. Unit	Bolus Dose Amt. LHL	Bolus Dose Amt. LSL	Bolus Dose Amt. USL	Bolus Dose Amt. UHL	Bolus Time LHL	Bolus Time LSL	Bolus Time USL	Bolus Time UHL	Bolus Dose Rate Dosing Unit
units			6000	10000			0:06		
units/ kg		0.1	0.15						
mg/kg			2			1:00			
mL				1000					

Source: With permission from Fairview Health Services, Minneapolis, Minnesota.

Table A-2. Bolus Dosing (cont'd)

Displayed Name	CCA Name	Med. Amount	Med. Unit	Diluent Amount	Diluent Unit	Bolus Enabled
L-asparaginase	Oncology		units	50	mL	
azacitidine	Oncology		mg	100	mL	
bendamustine	Oncology		mg	500	mL	
BEVACizumab over 30 min	Oncology		mg	100	mL	
BEVACizumab over 60 min	Oncology		mg	100	mL	
BEVACizumab over 90 min	Oncology		mg	100	mL	
bleomycin	Oncology		units	50	mL	
busulfan	Oncology	0.5	mg	1	mL	
CARBoplatin	Oncology		mg	100	mL	
CARBoplatin	Oncology		mg	250	mL	
CARBoplatin	Oncology		mg	500	mL	
CARBoplatin over 24 hr	Oncology		mg	1000	mL	
CARBoplatin desens	Oncology		mg	100	mL	
CARBoplatin desens	Oncology		mg	150	mL	
carmustine (BCNU)	Oncology		mg	250	mL	
CETuximab	Oncology	2	mg	1	mL	
chemotherapy infusion	Oncology				mL	
CISplatin	Oncology		mg	250	mL	
CISplatin	Oncology		mg	500	mL	
CISplatin	Oncology		mg	1000	mL	
CISplatin NO manitol	Oncology	1	mg	1	mL	

Bolus Dose Amt. Unit	Bolus Dose Amt. LHL	Bolus Dose Amt. LSL	Bolus Dose Amt. USL	Bolus Dose Amt. UHL	Bolus Time LHL	Bolus Time LSL	Bolus Time USL	Bolus Time UHL	Bolus Dose Rate Dosing Unit

Source: With permission from Fairview Health Services, Minneapolis, Minnesota.

Table A-2. Bolus Dosing (cont'd)

Displayed Name	CCA Name	Med. Amount	Med. Unit	Diluent Amount	Diluent Unit	Bolus Enabled
cladribine	Oncology		mg	250	mL	
clofarabine	Oncology	0.4	mg	1	mL	
cycloPHOSPHAMIDE	Oncology		mg	250	mL	
cycloPHOSPHAMIDE	Oncology		mg	500	mL	
CYTarabine (high dose)	Oncology		grams	250	mL	
CYTarabine over 1 hr	Oncology		mg	100	mL	
CYTarabine over 3 hr	Oncology		mg	250	mL	
CYTarabine continuous infusion	Oncology		mg	1000	mL	
dacarbazine	Oncology		mg	250	mL	
DAUNOrubicin	Oncology		mg	100	mL	
DAUNOrubicin liposomal	Oncology	1	mg	1	mL	
decitabine	Oncology		mg	100	mL	
decitabine	Oncology		mg	250	mL	
dexrazoxane (Totect)	Oncology		mg	1000	mL	
dexrazoxane (Zinecard)	Oncology		mg	100	mL	
DOCetaxel	Oncology		mg	250	mL	
DOCetaxel	Oncology		mg	500	mL	
DOXOrubicin over 1 hr	Oncology		mg	100	mL	
DOXOrubicin over 24 hr	Oncology		mg	1000	mL	
DOXOrubicin liposomal	Oncology		mg	250	mL	
DOXOrubicin liposomal	Oncology		mg	500	mL	

Source: With permission from Fairview Health Services, Minneapolis, Minnesota.

Bolus Dose Amt. Unit	Bolus Dose Amt. LHL	Bolus Dose Amt. LSL	Bolus Dose Amt. USL	Bolus Dose Amt. UHL	Bolus Time LHL	Bolus Time LSL	Bolus Time USL	Bolus Time UHL	Bolus Dose Rate Dosing Unit

Source: With permission from Fairview Health Services, Minneapolis, Minnesota.

Table A-2. Bolus Dosing (cont'd)

Displayed Name	CCA Name	Med. Amount	Med. Unit	Diluent Amount	Diluent Unit	Bolus Enabled
eculizumab	Oncology	600	mg	120	mL	
eculizumab	Oncology	900	mg	180	mL	
etoposide VP-16	Oncology		mg	250	mL	
etoposide VP-16	Oncology		mg	500	mL	
etoposide VP-16	Oncology		mg	1000	mL	
etoposide phosphate (Etopophos)	Oncology		mg	100	mL	
floxuridine	Oncology		mg	500	mL	
FLUdarabine	Oncology		mg	100	mL	
fluorouracil over 24 hr	Oncology		mg	1000	mL	
ganciclovir	Oncology		mg	100	mL	
gemcitabine	Oncology		grams	250	mL	
gemtuzumab	Oncology		mg	100	mL	
IDArubicin	Oncology		mg	100	mL	
ifosfamide	Oncology		grams	100	mL	
ifosfamide	Oncology		grams	250	mL	
ifosfamide	Oncology		grams	1000	mL	
ifosfamide + mesna	Oncology			1000	mL	
interferon alpha	Oncology		units	100	mL	
investigational chemo	Oncology		mg		mL	
irinotecan	Oncology		mg	250	mL	
irinotecan	Oncology		mg	500	mL	

Source: With permission from Fairview Health Services, Minneapolis, Minnesota.

Bolus Dose Amt. Unit	Bolus Dose Amt. LHL	Bolus Dose Amt. LSL	Bolus Dose Amt. USL	Bolus Dose Amt. UHL	Bolus Time LHL	Bolus Time LSL	Bolus Time USL	Bolus Time UHL	Bolus Dose Rate Dosing Unit

Source: With permission from Fairview Health Services, Minneapolis, Minnesota.

Table A-2. Bolus Dosing (cont'd)

Displayed Name	CCA Name	Med. Amount	Med. Unit	Diluent Amount	Diluent Unit	Bolus Enabled
ixabepilone	Oncology		mg	250	mL	
mesna intermittent	Oncology		mg	50	mL	
mesna cont infusion	Oncology		mg	1000	mL	
METHOTREXate/ sodium Bicarb	Oncology			500	mL	
METHOTREXate/ sodium bicarb	Oncology			1000	mL	
METHOTREXate	Oncology		mg	100	mL	
mitoxantrone	Oncology		mg	50	mL	
natalizumab	Oncology	300	mg	100	mL	
nelarabine	Oncology	5	mg	1	mL	
Other Drug	Oncology		Select on Infuser		mL	x
oxaliplatin	Oncology		mg	500	mL	
PACLitaxel over 1 hour	Oncology		mg	250	mL	
PACLitaxel over 3 hours	Oncology		mg	500	mL	
PACLitaxel over 24 hours	Oncology		mg	500	mL	
PACLitaxel prtn bd (abraxane)	Oncology	5	mg	1	mL	
pegaspargase	Oncology		units	100	mL	
pemetrexed	Oncology		mg	100	mL	
pentostatin	Oncology		mg	50	mL	
rasburicase	Oncology		mg	50	mL	
rituximab	Oncology	1	mg	1	mL	
streptozocin	Oncology		mg	100	mL	

Source: With permission from Fairview Health Services, Minneapolis, Minnesota.

Bolus Dose Amt. Unit	Bolus Dose Amt. LHL	Bolus Dose Amt. LSL	Bolus Dose Amt. USL	Bolus Dose Amt. UHL	Bolus Time LHL	Bolus Time LSL	Bolus Time USL	Bolus Time UHL	Bolus Dose Rate Dosing Unit

Source: With permission from Fairview Health Services, Minneapolis, Minnesota.

Table A-2. Bolus Dosing (cont'd)

Displayed Name	CCA Name	Med. Amount	Med. Unit	Diluent Amount	Diluent Unit	Bolus Enabled
TEMSIRolimus	Oncology		mg	250	mL	
teniposide	Oncology		mg	250	mL	
teniposide	Oncology		mg	500	mL	
teniposide	Oncology		mg	1000	mL	
thiotepa	Oncology		mg	50	mL	
thiotepa	Oncology		mg	100	mL	
thiotepa	Oncology		mg	250	mL	
topotecan	Oncology		mg	100	mL	
TRASTuzumab over 30 min	Oncology		mg	250	mL	
TRASTuzumab over 90 min	Oncology		mg	250	mL	
vinBLAStine-infuse via gravity	Oncology		mg	25	mL	
vinCRISTine	Oncology		mg	1000	mL	
vinCRIStine infuse via gravity	Oncology		mg	25	mL	
vinoRELBine infuse via gravity	Oncology		mg	25	mL	
zoledronic acid	Oncology		mg	100	mL	
IV fluid	Outpt Infu				mL	x
Premedication	Outpt Infu		mg		mL	
blood products	Outpt Infu				mL	
potassium chloride	Outpt Infu	10	mEq	100	mL	
potassium chloride	Outpt Infu	20	mEq	50	mL	
magnesium replacement	Outpt Infu	1	grams	50	mL	

Source: With permission from Fairview Health Services, Minneapolis, Minnesota.

Bolus Dose Amt. Unit	Bolus Dose Amt. LHL	Bolus Dose Amt. LSL	Bolus Dose Amt. USL	Bolus Dose Amt. UHL	Bolus Time LHL	Bolus Time LSL	Bolus Time USL	Bolus Time UHL	Bolus Dose Rate Dosing Unit
mL			1000						

Source: With permission from Fairview Health Services, Minneapolis, Minnesota.

Table A-2. Bolus Dosing (cont'd)

Displayed Name	CCA Name	Med. Amount	Med. Unit	Diluent Amount	Diluent Unit	Bolus Enabled
magnesium replacement	Outpt Infu		grams	100	mL	
antibiotic (except vancomycin)	Outpt Infu			50	mL	
antibiotic (except vancomycin)	Outpt Infu			100	mL	
antibiotic (except vancomycin)	Outpt Infu			150	mL	
antibiotic (except vancomycin)	Outpt Infu			250	mL	
antibiotic (except vancomycin)	Outpt Infu			500	mL	
vancomycin	Outpt Infu		mg		mL	
abatacept	Outpt Infu		mg	100	mL	
calcium CHLORide	Outpt Infu		grams	100	mL	
calcium GLUConate	Outpt Infu	1	grams	100	mL	
ferric gluconate	Outpt Infu	125	mg	100	mL	
ferric gluconate	Outpt Infu	250	mg	250	mL	
immune globulin-sucrose out pat	Outpt Infu				mL	
immune globulin-sucrose free op	Outpt Infu				mL	
infliximab	Outpt Infu		mg	250	mL	
iron dextran test dose	Outpt Infu	25	mg	50	mL	
iron dextran	Outpt Infu		mg	500	mL	
iron sucrose (Venofer)	Outpt Infu	200	mg	100	mL	
iron sucrose (Venofer)	Outpt Infu	500	mg	250	mL	
mannitol injection 20%	Outpt Infu	50	grams	250	mL	
mannitol injection 20%	Outpt Infu	100	grams	500	mL	

Source: With permission from Fairview Health Services, Minneapolis, Minnesota.

Bolus Dose Amt. Unit	Bolus Dose Amt. LHL	Bolus Dose Amt. LSL	Bolus Dose Amt. USL	Bolus Dose Amt. UHL	Bolus Time LHL	Bolus Time LSL	Bolus Time USL	Bolus Time UHL	Bolus Dose Rate Dosing Unit

Source: With permission from Fairview Health Services, Minneapolis, Minnesota.

Table A-2. Bolus Dosing (cont'd)

Displayed Name	CCA Name	Med. Amount	Med. Unit	Diluent Amount	Diluent Unit	Bolus Enabled
mannitol injection 25%	Outpt Infu	12.5	grams	50	mL	
mannitol injection 25%	Outpt Infu		grams		mL	
methylprednisolone	Outpt Infu		mg	100	mL	
Other Drug	Outpt Infu		Select on In- fuser		mL	x
pamidronate	Outpt Infu		mg	250	mL	
pamidronate	Outpt Infu		mg	500	mL	
pamidronate	Outpt Infu		mcg	1000	mL	
prolastin	Outpt Infu		mg		mL	
ranitidine intermit- tent	Outpt Infu	50	mg	50	mL	
thymoglobulin	Outpt Infu	50	mg	115	mL	
thymoglobulin	Outpt Infu	75	mg	173	mL	
thymoglobulin	Outpt Infu	100	mg	283	mL	
thymoglobulin-pe- ripheral	Outpt Infu		mg	500	mL	
zoledronic acid	Outpt Infu		mg	100	mL	
IV fluid	adultbmt				mL	x
calcium GLUConate	adultbmt	1	grams	100	mL	
cyclosporine	adultbmt		mg	100	mL	
cyclosporine	adultbmt		mg	150	mL	
cyclosporine	adultbmt		mg	250	mL	
cyclosporine drip BMT	adultbmt	250	mg	250	mL	
cyclosporine drip BMT	adultbmt	500	mg	250	mL	
filgrastim	adultbmt	15	mcg	1	mL	
foscarnet	adultbmt		mg		mL	
ganciclovir	adultbmt		mg	100	mL	

Source: With permission from Fairview Health Services, Minneapolis, Minnesota.

Bolus Dose Amt. Unit	Bolus Dose Amt. LHL	Bolus Dose Amt. LSL	Bolus Dose Amt. USL	Bolus Dose Amt. UHL	Bolus Time LHL	Bolus Time LSL	Bolus Time USL	Bolus Time UHL	Bolus Dose Rate Dosing Unit
mL			1000						

Source: With permission from Fairview Health Services, Minneapolis, Minnesota.

Table A-2. Bolus Dosing (cont'd)

Displayed Name	CCA Name	Med. Amount	Med. Unit	Diluent Amount	Diluent Unit	Bolus Enabled
lipids 20%	adultbmt	50	grams	250	mL	
lipids 20%	adultbmt	100	grams	500	mL	
magnesium replacement	adultbmt		grams		mL	
methylprednisolone	adultbmt		mg	100	mL	
phytonadione (vitamin K)	adultbmt		mg	50	mL	
potassium chloride	adultbmt	10	mEq	100	mL	
potassium chloride	adultbmt	20	mEq	50	mL	
potassium phosphate	adultbmt		mmol	500	mL	
potassium phosphate	adultbmt		mmol	250	mL	
sodium phosphate	adultbmt		mmol	250	mL	
sodium phosphate	adultbmt		mmol	500	mL	
TPN	adultbmt				mL	
3% sodium chloride	adultbmt				mL	
AMIODarone	adultbmt	500	mg	500	mL	x
AMIODarone	adultbmt	1500	mg	250	mL	x
antibiotic (except vancomycin)	adultbmt			50	mL	
antibiotic (except vancomycin)	adultbmt			100	mL	
antibiotic (except vancomycin)	adultbmt			150	mL	
antibiotic (except vancomycin)	adultbmt			250	mL	
antibiotic (except vancomycin)	adultbmt			500	mL	
antithymocyte globulin horse	adultbmt		grams	250	mL	
antithymocyte globulin horse	adultbmt		grams	500	mL	
antithymocyte globulin horse	adultbmt		mg	150	mL	
bumetanide ICU	adultbmt	25	mg	100	mL	x
chemo infusion	adultbmt				mL	
calcium CHLORide	adultbmt		grams	100	mL	
chlorpromazine	adultbmt	25	mg	50	mL	
chlorpromazine	adultbmt	50	mg	100	mL	

Source: With permission from Fairview Health Services, Minneapolis, Minnesota.

Bolus Dose Amt. Unit	Bolus Dose Amt. LHL	Bolus Dose Amt. LSL	Bolus Dose Amt. USL	Bolus Dose Amt. UHL	Bolus Time LHL	Bolus Time LSL	Bolus Time USL	Bolus Time UHL	Bolus Dose Rate Dosing Unit
mg				150	0:10		0:30		
mg				150	0:10		0:30		
mg				2					

Source: With permission from Fairview Health Services, Minneapolis, Minnesota.

Table A-2. Bolus Dosing (cont'd)

Displayed Name	CCA Name	Med. Amount	Med. Unit	Diluent Amount	Diluent Unit	Bolus Enabled
cidofovir	adultbmt		mg	100	mL	
dantrolene	adultbmt		mg		mL	
desmopressin	adultbmt		mcg	50	mL	
diltiazem	adultbmt	125	mg	125	mL	x
fentanyl	adultbmt	5	mg	100	mL	x
furosemide	adultbmt	100	mg	100	mL	x
HEParin	adultbmt	25000	units	250	mL	x
HYDROmorphone	adultbmt		mg		mL	x
immune globulin-sucrose	adultbmt				mL	
immune globulin-sucrose free	adultbmt				mL	
ketamine	adultbmt		mg		mL	x
leucovorin	adultbmt	10	mg	1	mL	
levetiracetam	adultbmt			100	mL	
lorazepam	adultbmt	50	mg	50	mL	x
metoclopramide	adultbmt		mg	50	mL	
midazolam	adultbmt	50	mg	50	mL	x
morphine	adultbmt		mg		mL	x
mycophenolate 500 mg dose	adultbmt	500	mg		mL	
mycophenolate 1000 mg dose	adultbmt	1000	mg		mL	
mycophenolate 1500 mg dose	adultbmt	1500	mg		mL	
octreotide	adultbmt	1250	mcg	250	mL	
ondansetron drip	adultbmt	50	mg	50	mL	
Other Drug	adultbmt		Select on Infuser		mL	x
PANtoprazole	adultbmt	80	mg	100	mL	
premedication	adultbmt		mg	50	mL	
rituximab	adultbmt	1	mg	1	mL	
sodium bicarbonate	adultbmt		mEq		mL	
tacrolimus	adultbmt	5	mg	250	mL	
thymoglobulin-BMT	adultbmt		mg	100	mL	
thymoglobulin-BMT	adultbmt		mg	150	mL	

Source: With permission from Fairview Health Services, Minneapolis, Minnesota.

Bolus Dose Amt. Unit	Bolus Dose Amt. LHL	Bolus Dose Amt. LSL	Bolus Dose Amt. USL	Bolus Dose Amt. UHL	Bolus Time LHL	Bolus Time LSL	Bolus Time USL	Bolus Time UHL	Bolus Dose Rate Dosing Unit
mg			35	60					
mcg									
mg			80						
units			6000	10000			0:06		
mg									
mg				10	0:03				
mg			4				0:02	0:05	
mg			4				0:02	0:05	
mg									

Source: With permission from Fairview Health Services, Minneapolis, Minnesota.

Table A-2. Bolus Dosing (cont'd)

Displayed Name	CCA Name	Med. Amount	Med. Unit	Diluent Amount	Diluent Unit	Bolus Enabled
thymoglobulin-BMT	adultbmt		mg	250	mL	
thymoglobulin-BMT	adultbmt		mg	500	mL	
vancomycin	adultbmt		mg		mL	
zoledronic acid	adultbmt		mg	100	mL	
Chemo over 30 min in ~50 mL	adultbmt			50	mL	
Chemo over 30 min in ~100 mL	adultbmt			100	mL	
Chemo over 30 min ~150 mL	adultbmt			150	mL	
Chemo over 30 min in ~250 mL	adultbmt			250	mL	
Chemo over 30 min in ~500 mL	adultbmt			500	mL	
chemo over 1 hour ~ 100 mL	adultbmt			100	mL	
chemo over 1 hour ~ 150 mL	adultbmt			150	mL	
chemo over 1 hour ~ 250 mL	adultbmt			250	mL	
Chemo over 1 hr in ~500 mL	adultbmt			500	mL	
Chemo over 2 hr in ~100 mL	adultbmt			100	mL	
Chemo over 2 hr in ~ 150mL	adultbmt			150	mL	
Chemo over 2 hr in ~ 250 mL	adultbmt			250	mL	
Chemo over 2 hr in ~ 500 mL	adultbmt			500	mL	
Chemo over 3 hr in ~ 250 mL	adultbmt			250	mL	
Chemo over 3 hr in ~ 500 mL	adultbmt			500	mL	
Chemo over 24 hr in ~1000 mL	adultbmt			1000	mL	
IV fluid	intermed				mL	x
blood products	intermed				mL	
antibiotic (except vancomycin)	intermed			50	mL	

Source: With permission from Fairview Health Services, Minneapolis, Minnesota.

Bolus Dose Amt. Unit	Bolus Dose Amt. LHL	Bolus Dose Amt. LSL	Bolus Dose Amt. USL	Bolus Dose Amt. UHL	Bolus Time LHL	Bolus Time LSL	Bolus Time USL	Bolus Time UHL	Bolus Dose Rate Dosing Unit
mL			1000						

Source: With permission from Fairview Health Services, Minneapolis, Minnesota.

Table A-2. Bolus Dosing (cont'd)

Displayed Name	CCA Name	Med. Amount	Med. Unit	Diluent Amount	Diluent Unit	Bolus Enabled
antibiotic (except vancomycin)	intermed			100	mL	
antibiotic (except vancomycin)	intermed			150	mL	
antibiotic (except vancomycin)	intermed			250	mL	
antibiotic (except vancomycin)	intermed			500	mL	
AMIODarone	intermed	500	mg	500	mL	x
AMIODarone	intermed	1500	mg	250	mL	x
diltiazem	intermed	125	mg	125	mL	x
HEParin	intermed	25000	units	250	mL	x
nitroGLYCERIN-IMC	intermed	50	mg	250	mL	
nitroGLYCERIN-IMC	intermed	200	mg	250	mL	
milrinone	intermed	20	mg	100	mL	x
furosemide	intermed	100	mg	100	mL	x
DOBUTamine-IMC	intermed	500	mg	250	mL	
DOBUTamine-IMC	intermed	1000	mg	250	mL	
DOPamine-IMC	intermed	400	mg	250	mL	
DOPamine-IMC	intermed	800	mg	250	mL	
esmolol	intermed	2000	mg	100	mL	x
potassium chloride	intermed	10	mEq	100	mL	
potassium chloride	intermed	20	mEq	50	mL	
TPN	intermed				mL	
lipids 20%	intermed	50	grams	250	mL	
lipids 20%	intermed	100	grams	500	mL	
magnesium replacement	intermed		grams		mL	
thymoglobulin	intermed	50	mg	115	mL	
thymoglobulin	intermed	75	mg	173	mL	
thymoglobulin	intermed	100	mg	283	mL	
thymoglobulin-peripheral	intermed		mg	500	mL	
immune globulin-sucrose	intermed				mL	
immune globulin-sucrose free	intermed				mL	
3% sodium chloride	intermed				mL	

Source: With permission from Fairview Health Services, Minneapolis, Minnesota.

Bolus Dose Amt. Unit	Bolus Dose Amt. LHL	Bolus Dose Amt. LSL	Bolus Dose Amt. USL	Bolus Dose Amt. UHL	Bolus Time LHL	Bolus Time LSL	Bolus Time USL	Bolus Time UHL	Bolus Dose Rate Dosing Unit
mg				150	0:10		0:30		
mg				150	0:10		0:30		
mg			35	60					
units			6000	10000			0:06		
mg			5						
mg			80						
mg			60						

Source: With permission from Fairview Health Services, Minneapolis, Minnesota.

Table A-2. Bolus Dosing (cont'd)

Displayed Name	CCA Name	Med. Amount	Med. Unit	Diluent Amount	Diluent Unit	Bolus Enabled
abciximab 80 kg or more	intermed	9	mg	250	mL	x
abciximab less than 80 kg	intermed	9	mg	250	mL	x
acetylcysteine-renal	intermed	600	mg	100	mL	
acetylcysteine-renal	intermed	1200	mg	100	mL	
alemtuzumab	intermed		mg	100	mL	
alteplase PE	intermed	100	mg	100	mL	x
alteplase stroke	intermed		mg		mL	x
argatroban-cath lab	intermed	250	mg	250	mL	
argatroban non-cath lab	intermed	250	mg	250	mL	
basiliximab	intermed		mg	50	mL	
BEVACizumab over 30 min	intermed		mg	100	mL	
BEVACizumab over 60 min	intermed		mg	100	mL	
BEVACizumab over 90 min	intermed		mg	100	mL	
bumetanide	intermed	25	mg	100	mL	x
calcium CHLORide	intermed		grams	100	mL	
calcium GLUConate	intermed	1	grams	100	mL	
chlorpromazine	intermed	25	mg	50	mL	
chlorpromazine	intermed	50	mg	100	mL	
conivaptan	intermed	20	mg	250	mL	x
cyclosporine drip-solid organ	intermed	250	mg	250	mL	
cyclosporine drip-solid organ	intermed	500	mg	250	mL	
daclizumab	intermed		mg	50	mL	
deferoxamine	intermed		mg	250	mL	
desmopressin	intermed		mcg	50	mL	
eptifibatide	intermed	200	mg	100	mL	x
ferric gluconate	intermed	125	mg	100	mL	
ferric gluconate	intermed	250	mg	250	mL	
foscarnet	intermed		mg		mL	
fosphenytoin	intermed		mg		mL	
ganciclovir	intermed		mg	100	mL	

Source: With permission from Fairview Health Services, Minneapolis, Minnesota.

Bolus Dose Amt. Unit	Bolus Dose Amt. LHL	Bolus Dose Amt. LSL	Bolus Dose Amt. USL	Bolus Dose Amt. UHL	Bolus Time LHL	Bolus Time LSL	Bolus Time USL	Bolus Time UHL	Bolus Dose Rate Dosing Unit
mg			50						
mg				20					
mg				10		1:00			
mg				9				0:01	
mg				2					
mg				20	0:30				
mg				22.6					

Source: With permission from Fairview Health Services, Minneapolis, Minnesota.

Table A-2. Bolus Dosing (cont'd)

Displayed Name	CCA Name	Med. Amount	Med. Unit	Diluent Amount	Diluent Unit	Bolus Enabled
infliximab	intermed		mg	250	mL	
iron dextran	intermed		mg	500	mL	
iron dextran test dose	intermed	25	mg	50	mL	
iron sucrose (Venofer)	intermed	200	mg	100	mL	
iron sucrose (Venofer)	intermed	500	mg	250	mL	
isoproterenol-mcg/kg/min dosing	intermed	1	mg	50	mL	
lepirudin	intermed	100	mg	250	mL	x
levetiracetam	intermed			100	mL	
mannitol injection 20%	intermed	50	grams	250	mL	
mannitol injection 20%	intermed	100	grams	500	mL	
mannitol injection 25%	intermed	12.5	grams	50	mL	
mannitol injection 25%	intermed		grams		mL	
methylprednisolone	intermed		mg	100	mL	
mycophenolate 500 mg dose	intermed	500	mg		mL	
mycophenolate 1000 mg dose	intermed	1000	mg		mL	
mycophenolate 1500 mg dose	intermed	1500	mg		mL	
naloxone	intermed	4	mg	100	mL	x
octreotide	intermed	1250	mcg	250	mL	
ondansetron drip	intermed	50	mg	50	mL	
Other Drug	intermed		Select on Infuser		mL	x
PANtoprazole	intermed	80	mg	100	mL	
phytonadione (vitamin K)	intermed		mg	50	mL	
potassium phosphate	intermed		mmol	250	mL	
potassium phosphate	intermed		mmol	500	mL	
rituximab	intermed	1	mg	1	mL	
sodium bicarbonate	intermed		mEq		mL	

Source: With permission from Fairview Health Services, Minneapolis, Minnesota.

Bolus Dose Amt. Unit	Bolus Dose Amt. LHL	Bolus Dose Amt. LSL	Bolus Dose Amt. USL	Bolus Dose Amt. UHL	Bolus Time LHL	Bolus Time LSL	Bolus Time USL	Bolus Time UHL	Bolus Dose Rate Dosing Unit
mg				44					
mg			2						

Source: With permission from Fairview Health Services, Minneapolis, Minnesota.

Table A-2. Bolus Dosing (cont'd)

Displayed Name	CCA Name	Med. Amount	Med. Unit	Diluent Amount	Diluent Unit	Bolus Enabled
sodium phosphate	intermed		mmol	250	mL	
sodium phosphate	intermed		mmol	500	mL	
tacrolimus	intermed	5	mg	250	mL	
tenecteplase	intermed	5	mg	500	mL	
valproate	intermed		mg	100	mL	
vancomycin	intermed		mg		mL	

Table A-3. Drug Properties

Displayed Name	CCA Name	Med. Amt.	Med. Unit	Diluent Amt.	Diluent Unit	High Risk
aminocaproic acid	ICU	5	grams	100	mL	
AMIODarone	ICU	500	mg	500	mL	
AMIODarone	ICU	1500	mg	250	mL	
cisatracurium	ICU	200	mg	100	mL	x
dexmedetomidine	ICU	200	mcg	50	mL	x
dexmedetomidine	ICU	400	mcg	100	mL	x
DOBUTamine	ICU	500	mg	250	mL	x
DOBUTamine	ICU	1000	mg	250	mL	x
DOPamine	ICU	400	mg	250	mL	x
DOPamine	ICU	800	mg	250	mL	x
EPInephrine	ICU	5	mg	250	mL	x
EPInephrine	ICU	16	mg	250	mL	x
EPInephrine-mcg/ kg/min dosing	ICU	5	mg	250	mL	x
EPInephrine-mcg/ kg/min dosing	ICU	16	mg	250	mL	x
esmolol	ICU	2000	mg	100	mL	
HEParin	ICU	25000	units	250	mL	x
isoproterenol	ICU	1	mg	50	mL	x
isoproterenol-mcg/ kg/min dosing	ICU	1	mg	50	mL	x
lidocaine	ICU	2	grams	250	mL	

Source: With permission from Fairview Health Services, Minneapolis, Minnesota.

Bolus Dose Amt. Unit	Bolus Dose Amt. LHL	Bolus Dose Amt. LSL	Bolus Dose Amt. USL	Bolus Dose Amt. UHL	Bolus Time LHL	Bolus Time LSL	Bolus Time USL	Bolus Time UHL	Bolus Dose Rate Dosing Unit

Basic Enabled	Piggyback Enabled	Intermittent Enabled	Multistep Enabled	Delivery at End of Infusion	Default KVO Rate (mL/hr)	Enable Piggyback & Bolus From Secondary
x				Continue		
x			x	Continue		
x			x	Continue		
x				Continue		
x				Continue		
x				Continue		
x				Continue		
x				Continue		
x				Continue		
x				Continue		
x				Continue		
x				Continue		
x				Continue		
x				Continue		
x				Continue		
x				Continue		
x				Continue		
x				Continue		
x				Continue		

Source: With permission from Fairview Health Services, Minneapolis, Minnesota.

Table A-3. Drug Properties (cont'd)

Displayed Name	CCA Name	Med. Amt.	Med. Unit	Diluent Amt.	Diluent Unit	High Risk
milrinone	ICU	20	mg	100	mL	x
NICARdipine	ICU	25	mg	250	mL	x
NICARdipine	ICU	100	mg	250	mL	x
nitroGLYCERIN	ICU	50	mg	250	mL	x
nitroGLYCERIN	ICU	200	mg	250	mL	x
nitroGLYCERIN-mcg/ kg/min dosing	ICU	50	mg	250	mL	x
nitroGLYCERIN-mcg/ kg/min dosing	ICU	200	mg	250	mL	x
nitroPRUSSide	ICU	100	mg	250	mL	x
nitroPRUSSide	ICU	400	mg	250	mL	x
NOREPInephrine	ICU	8	mg	250	mL	x
NOREPInephrine	ICU	16	mg	250	mL	x
NOREPInephrine-mcg/kg/min dosing	ICU	8	mg	250	mL	x
NOREPInephrine-mcg/kg/min dosing	ICU	16	mg	250	mL	x
phenylephrine	ICU	50	mg	250	mL	x
phenylephrine-mcg/ kg/min dosing	ICU	50	mg	250	mL	x
phenylephrine-mcg/ kg/min dosing	ICU	200	mg	250	mL	x
propofol	ICU	1000	mg	100	mL	x
vasopressin	ICU	100	units	100	mL	x
vecuronium	ICU	50	mg	50	mL	x
IV fluid	ICU				mL	
23.4% Sodium Chloride	ICU			30	mL	x
3% sodium chloride	ICU				mL	x
abciximab less than 80 kg	ICU	9	mg	250	mL	x
abciximab 80 kg or more	ICU	9	mg	250	mL	x
acetylcysteine Step 1	ICU		grams	200	mL	
acetylcysteine Step 2	ICU		grams	500	mL	
acetylcysteine Step 3	ICU		grams	1000	mL	
acetylcysteine-renal	ICU	600	mg	100	mL	
acetylcysteine-renal	ICU	1200	mg	100	mL	

Source: With permission from Fairview Health Services, Minneapolis, Minnesota.

Basic Enabled	Piggyback Enabled	Intermittent Enabled	Multistep Enabled	Delivery at End of Infusion	Default KVO Rate (mL/hr)	Enable Piggyback & Bolus From Secondary
x				Continue		
x				Continue		
x				Continue		
x				Continue		
x				Continue		
x				Continue		
x				Continue		
x				Continue		
x				Continue		
x				Continue		
x				Continue		
x				Continue		
x				Continue		
x				Continue		
x				Continue		
x				Continue		
x				Continue		
x				Continue		
x				Continue		
x	x		x	KVO	10	x
x				KVO	10	
x				KVO	10	
x				Continue		
x				Continue		
x				KVO	10	
x				KVO	10	
x				Continue		
x	x			KVO	10	
x	x			KVO	10	

Source: With permission from Fairview Health Services, Minneapolis, Minnesota.

Table A-3. Drug Properties [cont'd]

Displayed Name	CCA Name	Med. Amt.	Med. Unit	Diluent Amt.	Diluent Unit	High Risk
alemtuzumab	ICU		mg	100	mL	x
alprostadil	ICU	1	mg	100	mL	
alteplase PE	ICU	100	mg	100	mL	x
alteplase-rad	ICU	1	mg	100	mL	x
alteplase stroke	ICU		mg		mL	x
antibiotic (except vancomycin)	ICU			50	mL	
antibiotic (except vancomycin)	ICU			100	mL	
antibiotic (except vancomycin)	ICU			150	mL	
antibiotic (except vancomycin)	ICU			250	mL	
antibiotic (except vancomycin)	ICU			500	mL	
antithymocyte globulin horse	ICU		mg	50	mL	
antithymocyte globulin horse	ICU		mg	100	mL	
antithymocyte globulin horse	ICU		mg	150	mL	
antithymocyte globulin horse	ICU		grams	250	mL	
antithymocyte globulin horse	ICU		grams	500	mL	
argatroban non-cath lab	ICU	250	mg	250	mL	x
argatroban-cath lab	ICU	250	mg	250	mL	x
basiliximab	ICU		mg	50	mL	
BEVACizumab over 30 min	ICU		mg	100	mL	x
BEVACizumab over 60 min	ICU		mg	100	mL	x
BEVACizumab over 90 min	ICU		mg	100	mL	x
bivalirudin non-cath lab	ICU	250	mg	50	mL	x
bivalirudin-cath lab	ICU	250	mg	50	mL	x
bumetanide ICU	ICU	25	mg	100	mL	
calcium CHLORide	ICU		grams	100	mL	

Source: With permission from Fairview Health Services, Minneapolis, Minnesota.

Basic Enabled	Piggyback Enabled	Intermittent Enabled	Multistep Enabled	Delivery at End of Infusion	Default KVO Rate (mL/hr)	Enable Piggyback & Bolus From Secondary
x	x			KVO	10	
x				Continue		
x				Continue		
x				KVO	10	
x				Continue		
x	x			KVO	10	
x	x			KVO	10	
x	x			KVO	10	
x	x			KVO	10	
x	x			KVO	10	
x	x		x	KVO	10	
x	x		x	KVO	10	
x	x		x	KVO	10	
x	x		x	KVO	10	
x	x		x	KVO	10	
x				Continue		
x				Continue		
x				Continue		
x	x			KVO	10	
x	x			KVO	10	
x	x			KVO	10	x
x				Continue		
x				Continue		
x				Continue		
x	x			KVO	10	

Source: With permission from Fairview Health Services, Minneapolis, Minnesota.

Table A-3. Drug Properties (cont'd)

Displayed Name	CCA Name	Med. Amt.	Med. Unit	Diluent Amt.	Diluent Unit	High Risk
calcium GLUConate	ICU	1	grams	100	mL	
chlorpromazine	ICU	25	mg	50	mL	
chlorpromazine	ICU	50	mg	100	mL	
cidofovir	ICU		mg	100	mL	
clevidipine	ICU	25	mg	50	mL	
conivaptan	ICU	20	mg	250	mL	
cyclosporine	ICU		mg	100	mL	
cyclosporine	ICU		mg	150	mL	
cyclosporine	ICU		mg	250	mL	
cyclosporine drip BMT	ICU	250	mg	250	mL	
cyclosporine drip BMT	ICU	500	mg	250	mL	
cyclosporine drip-solid organ	ICU	250	mg	250	mL	
cyclosporine drip-solid organ	ICU	500	mg	250	mL	
daclizumab	ICU		mg	50	mL	
dantrolene	ICU		mg		mL	
deferoxamine	ICU		mg	250	mL	
desmopressin	ICU		mcg	50	mL	
echo-DOBUTamine	ICU	500	mg	250	mL	x
diltiazem	ICU	125	mg	125	mL	
drotrecogin alfa (xigris)	ICU	10	mg	100	mL	x
drotrecogin alfa (xigris)	ICU	20	mg	200	mL	x
eptifibatide	ICU	200	mg	100	mL	x
fentanyl	ICU	5	mg	100	mL	x
ferric gluconate	ICU	125	mg	100	mL	
ferric gluconate	ICU	250	mg	250	mL	
foscarnet	ICU		mg		mL	
fosphenytoin	ICU		mg		mL	
furosemide	ICU	100	mg	100	mL	
ganciclovir	ICU		mg	100	mL	x
HYDROmorphone	ICU		mg		mL	x

Source: With permission from Fairview Health Services, Minneapolis, Minnesota.

Basic Enabled	Piggyback Enabled	Intermittent Enabled	Multistep Enabled	Delivery at End of Infusion	Default KVO Rate (mL/hr)	Enable Piggyback & Bolus From Secondary
x	x			KVO	10	
x	x			KVO	10	
x	x			KVO	10	
x	x			KVO	10	
x				Continue		
x				Continue		
x	x			KVO	10	
x	x			KVO	10	
x	x			KVO	10	
x				Continue		
x				Continue		
x				Continue		
x				Continue		
x	x			KVO	10	
x	x			KVO	10	
x	x			KVO	10	
x	x			KVO	10	
x			x	Continue		
x				Continue		
x				Continue		
x				Continue		
x				Continue		
x	x			Continue		
x	x			KVO	10	
x	x			KVO	10	
x				KVO	10	
x				KVO	10	
x				Continue		
x	x			KVO	10	
x	x			Continue		

Source: With permission from Fairview Health Services, Minneapolis, Minnesota.

Table A-3. Drug Properties (cont'd)

Displayed Name	CCA Name	Med. Amt.	Med. Unit	Diluent Amt.	Diluent Unit	High Risk
immune globulin-sucrose	ICU				mL	
immune globulin-sucrose free	ICU				mL	
infliximab	ICU		mg	250	mL	
insulin-ICU	ICU	50	units	50	mL	x
iron dextran test dose	ICU	25	mg	50	mL	
iron dextran	ICU		mg	500	mL	
iron sucrose (Venofer)	ICU	200	mg	100	mL	
iron sucrose (Venofer)	ICU	500	mg	250	mL	
ketamine	ICU		mg		mL	x
labetalol	ICU	250	mg	50	mL	
lepirudin	ICU	100	mg	250	mL	x
leucovorin	ICU	10	mg	1	mL	
levetiracetam	ICU			100	mL	
lipids 20%	ICU	50	grams	250	mL	
lipids anesthetic overdose	ICU	50	grams	250	mL	
lorazepam	ICU	50	mg	50	mL	x
lorazepam	ICU	100	mg	100	mL	x
magnesium replacement	ICU		grams		mL	
methylprednisolone	ICU		mg	100	mL	
methylpred INF spinal cord	ICU		mg	500	mL	
methylpred bolus spinal cord	ICU		mg	100	mL	
metoclopramide	ICU		mg	50	mL	
midazolam	ICU	100	mg	100	mL	x
morphine	ICU		mg		mL	x
mycophenolate 500 mg dose	ICU	500	mg		mL	
mycophenolate 1000 mg dose	ICU	1000	mg		mL	
mycophenolate 1500 mg dose	ICU	1500	mg		mL	

Source: With permission from Fairview Health Services, Minneapolis, Minnesota.

Basic Enabled	Piggyback Enabled	Intermittent Enabled	Multistep Enabled	Delivery at End of Infusion	Default KVO Rate (mL/hr)	Enable Piggyback & Bolus From Secondary
x				KVO	10	
x				KVO	10	
x	x			KVO	10	
x				Continue		
x	x			KVO	10	
x	x			KVO	10	
x	x			KVO	10	
x	x			KVO	10	
x				Continue		
x				Continue		
x				Continue		
x	x		x	KVO	10	x
x	x			KVO	10	
x				KVO	10	
x	x			KVO	10	
x				Continue		
x				Continue		
x	x			KVO	10	
x	x			KVO	10	
x				Continue		
x	x			KVO	10	
x	x		x	KVO	10	x
x				Continue		
x	x			Continue		
x				KVO	10	
x				KVO	10	
x				KVO	10	

Source: With permission from Fairview Health Services, Minneapolis, Minnesota.

Table A-3. Drug Properties (cont'd)

Displayed Name	CCA Name	Med. Amt.	Med. Unit	Diluent Amt.	Diluent Unit	High Risk
naloxone	ICU	4	mg	100	mL	
nesiritide	ICU	1.5	mg	250	mL	
octreotide	ICU	1250	mcg	250	mL	
ondansetron drip	ICU	50	mg	50	mL	
Other Drug	ICU		Select on In-fuser		mL	
PANtoprazole	ICU	80	mg	100	mL	
PenTobarbital	ICU	2000	mg	250	mL	x
PHenobarbital	ICU	2000	mg	250	mL	x
phenytoin	ICU		mg		mL	
phytonadione (vitamin K)	ICU		mg	50	mL	
potassium chloride	ICU	10	mEq	100	mL	
potassium chloride	ICU	20	mEq	50	mL	
potassium phosphate	ICU		mmol	250	mL	
potassium phosphate	ICU		mmol	500	mL	
procainamide	ICU	2	grams	250	mL	
rituximab	ICU	1	mg	1	mL	x
rocuronium	ICU	500	mg	250	mL	x
sodium bicarbonate	ICU		mEq		mL	
sodium phosphate	ICU		mmol	250	mL	
sodium phosphate	ICU		mmol	500	mL	
tacrolimus	ICU	5	mg	250	mL	
tenecteplase	ICU	5	mg	500	mL	x
thymoglobulin	ICU	50	mg	115	mL	
thymoglobulin	ICU	75	mg	173	mL	
thymoglobulin	ICU	100	mg	283	mL	
thymoglobulin-peripheral	ICU		mg	500	mL	
TPN	ICU				mL	
valproate	ICU		mg	100	mL	
vancomycin	ICU		mg		mL	
zoledronic acid	ICU		mg	100	mL	
IV fluid	MedSurg				mL	
blood products	MedSurg				mL	x

Source: With permission from Fairview Health Services, Minneapolis, Minnesota.

Basic Enabled	Piggyback Enabled	Intermittent Enabled	Multistep Enabled	Delivery at End of Infusion	Default KVO Rate (mL/hr)	Enable Piggyback & Bolus From Secondary
x				Continue		
x				Continue		
x				Continue		
x	x			KVO	10	
x	x	x	x	KVO	1	x
x	x			Continue		
x				Continue		
x				Continue		
x	x			KVO	10	
x	x			KVO	10	
x	x			KVO	10	
x	x			KVO	10	
x	x			KVO	10	
x	x			KVO	10	
x				Continue		
x	x		x	KVO	10	
x	x			Continue		
x	x			KVO	10	
x	x			KVO	10	
x	x			KVO	10	
x				Continue		
x	x			KVO	10	
x	x			KVO	10	
x	x			KVO	10	
x	x			KVO	10	
x	x			KVO	10	
x			x	KVO	10	x
x	x			KVO	10	
x	x			KVO	10	
x	x			KVO	10	
x	x		x	KVO	10	x
x				KVO	10	

Source: With permission from Fairview Health Services, Minneapolis, Minnesota.

Table A-3. Drug Properties (cont'd)

Displayed Name	CCA Name	Med. Amt.	Med. Unit	Diluent Amt.	Diluent Unit	High Risk
antibiotic (except vancomycin)	MedSurg			50	mL	
antibiotic (except vancomycin)	MedSurg			100	mL	
antibiotic (except vancomycin)	MedSurg			150	mL	
antibiotic (except vancomycin)	MedSurg			250	mL	
antibiotic (except vancomycin)	MedSurg			500	mL	
vancomycin	MedSurg		mg		mL	
potassium chloride	MedSurg	10	mEq	100	mL	
potassium chloride	MedSurg	20	mEq	50	mL	
magnesium replacement	MedSurg		grams		mL	
TPN	MedSurg				mL	
lipids 20%	MedSurg	50	grams	250	mL	
lipids 20%	MedSurg	100	grams	500	mL	
HEParin	MedSurg	25000	units	250	mL	x
acetylcysteine-renal	MedSurg	600	mg	100	mL	
acetylcysteine-renal	MedSurg	1200	mg	100	mL	
alemtuzumab	MedSurg		mg	100	mL	x
alteplase stroke	MedSurg		mg		mL	x
alteplase PE	MedSurg	100	mg	100	mL	x
alteplase-rad	MedSurg	12.5	mg	50	mL	x
AMIODarone	MedSurg	500	mg	500	mL	
argatroban non-cath lab	MedSurg	250	mg	250	mL	x
basiliximab	MedSurg		mg	50	mL	
BEVACizumab over 30 min	MedSurg		mg	100	mL	x
BEVACizumab over 60 min	MedSurg		mg	100	mL	x
BEVACizumab over 90 min	MedSurg		mg	100	mL	x
bumetanide	MedSurg	25	mg	100	mL	
calcium CHLORide	MedSurg		grams	100	mL	
calcium GLUConate	MedSurg	1	grams	100	mL	

Source: With permission from Fairview Health Services, Minneapolis, Minnesota.

Basic Enabled	Piggyback Enabled	Intermittent Enabled	Multistep Enabled	Delivery at End of Infusion	Default KVO Rate (mL/hr)	Enable Piggyback & Bolus From Secondary
x	x			KVO	10	
x	x			KVO	10	
x	x			KVO	10	
x	x			KVO	10	
x	x			KVO	10	
x	x			KVO	10	
x	x			KVO	10	
x	x			KVO	10	
x	x			KVO	10	
x			x	KVO	10	x
x				KVO	10	
x				KVO	10	
x				Continue		
x	x			KVO	10	
x	x			KVO	10	
x	x			KVO	10	
x				Continue		
x				Continue		
x				KVO	10	
x			x	Continue		
x				Continue		
x				Continue		
x	x			KVO	10	
x	x			KVO	10	
x	x			KVO	10	x
x				Continue		x
x	x			KVO	10	
x	x			KVO	10	

Source: With permission from Fairview Health Services, Minneapolis, Minnesota.

Table A-3. Drug Properties (cont'd)

Displayed Name	CCA Name	Med. Amt.	Med. Unit	Diluent Amt.	Diluent Unit	High Risk
chlorpromazine	MedSurg	25	mg	50	mL	
chlorpromazine	MedSurg	50	mg	100	mL	
conivaptan	MedSurg	20	mg	250	mL	
cyclosporine drip-solid organ	MedSurg	250	mg	250	mL	
cyclosporine drip-solid organ	MedSurg	500	mg	250	mL	
daclizumab	MedSurg		mg	50	mL	
deferoxamine	MedSurg		mg	250	mL	
desmopressin	MedSurg		mcg	50	mL	
diltiazem	MedSurg	125	mg	125	mL	
ferric gluconate	MedSurg	125	mg	100	mL	
ferric gluconate	MedSurg	250	mg	250	mL	
foscarnet	MedSurg		mg		mL	
fosphenytoin	MedSurg		mg		mL	
furosemide	MedSurg	100	mg	100	mL	
ganciclovir	MedSurg		mg	100	mL	x
immune globulin-sucrose	MedSurg				mL	
immune globulin-sucrose free	MedSurg				mL	
infliximab	MedSurg		mg	250	mL	
insulin	MedSurg	50	units	50	mL	x
iron dextran test dose	MedSurg	25	mg	50	mL	
iron dextran	MedSurg		mg	500	mL	
iron sucrose (Venofer)	MedSurg	200	mg	100	mL	
iron sucrose (Venofer)	MedSurg	500	mg	250	mL	
lepirudin	MedSurg	100	mg	250	mL	x
levetiracetam	MedSurg			100	mL	
mannitol injection 20%	MedSurg	50	grams	250	mL	
mannitol injection 20%	MedSurg	100	grams	500	mL	
mannitol injection 25%	MedSurg	12.5	grams	50	mL	

Source: With permission from Fairview Health Services, Minneapolis, Minnesota.

Basic Enabled	Piggyback Enabled	Intermittent Enabled	Multistep Enabled	Delivery at End of Infusion	Default KVO Rate (mL/hr)	Enable Piggyback & Bolus From Secondary
x	x			KVO	10	
x	x			KVO	10	
x				Continue		
x				Continue		
x				Continue		
x	x			KVO	10	
x	x			KVO	10	
x	x			KVO	10	
x				Continue		
x	x			KVO	10	
x	x			KVO	10	
x				KVO	10	
x				KVO	10	
x				Continue		
x	x			KVO	10	
x				KVO	10	
x				KVO	10	
x	x			KVO	10	
x				Continue		
x	x			KVO	10	
x	x			KVO	10	
x	x			KVO	10	
x	x			KVO	10	
x				Continue		
x	x			KVO	10	
x				KVO	10	
x				KVO	10	
x				KVO	10	

Source: With permission from Fairview Health Services, Minneapolis, Minnesota.

Table A-3. Drug Properties (cont'd)

Displayed Name	CCA Name	Med. Amt.	Med. Unit	Diluent Amt.	Diluent Unit	High Risk
mannitol injection 25%	MedSurg		grams		mL	
metoclopramide	MedSurg		mg	50	mL	
methylprednisolone	MedSurg		mg	100	mL	
mycophenolate 500 mg dose	MedSurg	500	mg		mL	
mycophenolate 1000 mg dose	MedSurg	1000	mg		mL	
mycophenolate 1500 mg dose	MedSurg	1500	mg		mL	
naloxone	MedSurg	4	mg	100	mL	
octreotide	MedSurg	1250	mcg	250	mL	
ondansetron drip	MedSurg	50	mg	50	mL	
Other Drug	MedSurg		Select on Infuser		mL	
PANtoprazole	MedSurg	80	mg	100	mL	
phytonadione (vitamin K)	MedSurg		mg	50	mL	
potassium phosphate	MedSurg		mmol	250	mL	
potassium phosphate	MedSurg		mmol	500	mL	
rituximab	MedSurg	1	mg	1	mL	x
sodium bicarbonate	MedSurg		mEq		mL	
1.5% sodium chloride	MedSurg			1000	mL	x
3% sodium chloride	MedSurg				mL	x
sodium phosphate	MedSurg		mmol	250	mL	
sodium phosphate	MedSurg		mmol	500	mL	
tacrolimus	MedSurg	5	mg	250	mL	
thymoglobulin	MedSurg	50	mg	115	mL	
thymoglobulin	MedSurg	75	mg	173	mL	
thymoglobulin	MedSurg	100	mg	283	mL	
thymoglobulin-peripheral	MedSurg		mg	500	mL	
valproate	MedSurg		mg	100	mL	
IV fluid	OB				mL	
oxytocin-labor	OB	20	units	1000	mL	
oxytocin-postpartum	OB	20	units	1000	mL	
oxytocin-postpartum	OB	40	units	1000	mL	

Source: With permission from Fairview Health Services, Minneapolis, Minnesota.

Basic Enabled	Piggyback Enabled	Intermittent Enabled	Multistep Enabled	Delivery at End of Infusion	Default KVO Rate (mL/hr)	Enable Piggyback & Bolus From Secondary
x				KVO	10	
x	x		x	KVO	10	x
x	x			KVO	10	
x				KVO	10	
x				KVO	10	
x				KVO	10	
x				Continue		
x				Continue		
x	x			KVO	10	
x	x	x	x	KVO	1	x
x	x			Continue		
x	x			KVO	10	
x	x			KVO	10	
x	x			KVO	10	
x	x		x	KVO	10	
x	x			KVO	10	
x				Continue		
x				KVO	10	
x	x			KVO	10	
x	x			KVO	10	
x				Continue		
x	x			KVO	10	
x	x			KVO	10	
x	x			KVO	10	
x	x			KVO	10	
x	x			KVO	10	
x	x		x	KVO	10	x
x	x			Continue		
x	x			Continue		
x	x			Continue		

Source: With permission from Fairview Health Services, Minneapolis, Minnesota.

Table A-3. Drug Properties (cont'd)

Displayed Name	CCA Name	Med. Amt.	Med. Unit	Diluent Amt.	Diluent Unit	High Risk
magnesium sulfate infusion	OB	20	grams	500	mL	
magnesium seizure	OB	2	grams	50	mL	
magnesium seizure	OB	4	grams	50	mL	x
antibiotic (except vancomycin)	OB			50	mL	
antibiotic (except vancomycin)	OB			100	mL	
antibiotic (except vancomycin)	OB			150	mL	
antibiotic (except vancomycin)	OB			250	mL	
antibiotic (except vancomycin)	OB			500	mL	
vancomycin	OB		mg		mL	
blood products	OB				mL	x
HEParin	OB	25000	units	250	mL	x
insulin-OB	OB	50	units	50	mL	x
TPN	OB				mL	
lipids 20%	OB	50	grams	250	mL	
lipids 20%	OB	100	grams	500	mL	
potassium chloride	OB	10	mEq	100	mL	
hetastarch (Hespan)	OB			500	mL	
Other Drug	OB		Select on In- fuser		mL	
fosphenytoin	OB		mg		mL	
zidovudine	OB		mg		mL	
IV fluid	Oncology				mL	
premedication	Oncology		mg	50	mL	
premedication	Oncology		mg	100	mL	
premedication	Oncology		mg	150	mL	
ALDESleukin	Oncology		Million Units	50	mL	x
alemtuzumab	Oncology		mg	100	mL	x
amifostine	Oncology		mg	50	mL	x
antithymocyte globu- lin horse	Oncology		mg	50	mL	

Source: With permission from Fairview Health Services, Minneapolis, Minnesota.

Basic Enabled	Piggyback Enabled	Intermittent Enabled	Multistep Enabled	Delivery at End of Infusion	Default KVO Rate (mL/hr)	Enable Piggyback & Bolus From Secondary
x				Continue		
x	x			KVO	10	
x	x			KVO	10	
x	x			KVO	10	
x	x			KVO	10	
x	x			KVO	10	
x	x			KVO	10	
x	x			KVO	10	
x	x			KVO	10	
x				KVO	10	
x				Continue		
x				Continue		
x				Continue		x
x				KVO	10	
x				KVO	10	
x	x			KVO	10	
x				KVO	10	
x	x	x	x	KVO	1	x
x				KVO	10	
x	x			KVO	10	
x	x		x	KVO	10	x
x	x			KVO	10	
x	x			KVO	10	
x	x			KVO	10	
x	x			KVO	10	
x	x			KVO	10	
x	x			KVO	10	
x	x		x	KVO	10	

Source: With permission from Fairview Health Services, Minneapolis, Minnesota.

Table A-3. Drug Properties (cont'd)

Displayed Name	CCA Name	Med. Amt.	Med. Unit	Diluent Amt.	Diluent Unit	High Risk
antithymocyte globulin horse	Oncology		mg	100	mL	
antithymocyte globulin horse	Oncology		mg	150	mL	
antithymocyte globulin horse	Oncology		grams	250	mL	
antithymocyte globulin horse	Oncology		grams	500	mL	
arsenic trioxide	Oncology		mg	250	mL	x
L-asparaginase	Oncology		units	50	mL	x
azacitidine	Oncology		mg	100	mL	x
bendamustine	Oncology		mg	500	mL	x
BEVACizumab over 30 min	Oncology		mg	100	mL	x
BEVACizumab over 60 min	Oncology		mg	100	mL	x
BEVACizumab over 90 min	Oncology		mg	100	mL	x
bleomycin	Oncology		units	50	mL	x
busulfan	Oncology	0.5	mg	1	mL	x
CARBoplatin	Oncology		mg	100	mL	x
CARBoplatin	Oncology		mg	250	mL	x
CARBoplatin	Oncology		mg	500	mL	x
CARBoplatin over 24 hr	Oncology		mg	1000	mL	x
CARBoplatin desens	Oncology		mg	100	mL	x
CARBoplatin desens	Oncology		mg	150	mL	x
carmustine (BCNU)	Oncology		mg	250	mL	x
CETuximab	Oncology	2	mg	1	mL	x
chemotherapy infusion	Oncology				mL	x
CISplatin	Oncology		mg	250	mL	x
CISplatin	Oncology		mg	500	mL	x
CISplatin	Oncology		mg	1000	mL	x
CISplatin NO manitol	Oncology	1	mg	1	mL	x
cladribine	Oncology		mg	250	mL	x
clofarabine	Oncology	0.4	mg	1	mL	x
cycloPHOSPHAMIDE	Oncology		mg	250	mL	x

Source: With permission from Fairview Health Services, Minneapolis, Minnesota.

Basic Enabled	Piggyback Enabled	Intermittent Enabled	Multistep Enabled	Delivery at End of Infusion	Default KVO Rate (mL/hr)	Enable Piggyback & Bolus From Secondary
x	x		x	KVO	10	
x	x		x	KVO	10	
x	x		x	KVO	10	
x	x		x	KVO	10	
x	x			KVO	10	
x	x			KVO	10	
x	x			KVO	10	
x				KVO	10	
x	x			KVO	10	
x	x			KVO	10	
x	x			KVO	10	x
x	x			KVO	10	
x	x			KVO	10	
x	x			KVO	10	
x	x			KVO	10	
x	x			KVO	10	
x	x			KVO	10	
x	x			KVO	10	
x	x			KVO	10	
x	x			KVO	10	
x	x			KVO	10	
x	x			KVO	10	
x	x			KVO	10	x
x				KVO	10	x
x				KVO	10	x
x	x			KVO	10	x
x	x			KVO	10	x
x	x			KVO	10	
x				KVO	10	

Source: With permission from Fairview Health Services, Minneapolis, Minnesota.

Table A-3. Drug Properties (cont'd)

Displayed Name	CCA Name	Med. Amt.	Med. Unit	Diluent Amt.	Diluent Unit	High Risk
cycloPHOSPHAMIDE	Oncology		mg	500	mL	x
CYTarabine (high dose)	Oncology		grams	250	mL	x
CYTarabine over 1 hr	Oncology		mg	100	mL	x
CYTarabine over 3 hr	Oncology		mg	250	mL	x
CYTarabine continuous infusion	Oncology		mg	1000	mL	x
dacarbazine	Oncology		mg	250	mL	x
DAUNOrubicin	Oncology		mg	100	mL	x
DAUNOrubicin liposomal	Oncology	1	mg	1	mL	x
decitabine	Oncology		mg	100	mL	x
decitabine	Oncology		mg	250	mL	x
dexrazoxane (Totect)	Oncology		mg	1000	mL	x
dexrazoxane (Zinecard)	Oncology		mg	100	mL	x
DOCetaxel	Oncology		mg	250	mL	x
DOCetaxel	Oncology		mg	500	mL	x
DOXOrubicin over 1 hr	Oncology		mg	100	mL	x
DOXOrubicin over 24 hr	Oncology		mg	1000	mL	x
DOXOrubicin liposomal	Oncology		mg	250	mL	x
DOXOrubicin liposomal	Oncology		mg	500	mL	x
eculizumab	Oncology	600	mg	120	mL	
eculizumab	Oncology	900	mg	180	mL	
etoposide VP-16	Oncology		mg	250	mL	x
etoposide VP-16	Oncology		mg	500	mL	x
etoposide VP-16	Oncology		mg	1000	mL	x
etoposide phosphate (Etopophos)	Oncology		mg	100	mL	x
floxuridine	Oncology		mg	500	mL	x
FLUdarabine	Oncology		mg	100	mL	x
fluorouracil over 24 hr	Oncology		mg	1000	mL	x
ganciclovir	Oncology		mg	100	mL	x

Source: With permission from Fairview Health Services, Minneapolis, Minnesota.

Basic Enabled	Piggyback Enabled	Intermittent Enabled	Multistep Enabled	Delivery at End of Infusion	Default KVO Rate (mL/hr)	Enable Piggyback & Bolus From Secondary
x				KVO	10	
x	x			KVO	10	
x	x			KVO	10	
x	x			KVO	10	
x	x			Continue		
x				KVO	10	
x	x			KVO	10	
x	x			KVO	10	
x	x			KVO	10	
x	x			KVO	10	
x				KVO	10	
x				KVO	10	
x	x			KVO	10	
x				KVO	10	
x	x			KVO	10	
x	x			Continue		
x	x			KVO	10	
x				KVO	10	
x	x			KVO	10	
x	x			KVO	10	
x				KVO	10	
x				KVO	10	
x				KVO	10	
x	x			KVO	10	
x				KVO	10	
x	x			KVO	10	
x	x			Continue		
x	x			KVO	10	

Source: With permission from Fairview Health Services, Minneapolis, Minnesota.

Table A-3. Drug Properties (cont'd)

Displayed Name	CCA Name	Med. Amt.	Med. Unit	Diluent Amt.	Diluent Unit	High Risk
gemcitabine	Oncology		grams	250	mL	x
gemtuzumab	Oncology		mg	100	mL	x
IDArubicin	Oncology		mg	100	mL	x
ifosfamide	Oncology		grams	100	mL	x
ifosfamide	Oncology		grams	250	mL	x
ifosfamide	Oncology		grams	1000	mL	x
ifosfamide + mesna	Oncology			1000	mL	x
interferon alpha	Oncology		units	100	mL	x
investigational chemo	Oncology		mg		mL	x
irinotecan	Oncology		mg	250	mL	x
irinotecan	Oncology		mg	500	mL	x
ixabepilone	Oncology		mg	250	mL	x
mesna intermittent	Oncology		mg	50	mL	
mesna cont infusion	Oncology		mg	1000	mL	
METHOTREXate/ sodium bicarb	Oncology			500	mL	x
METHOTREXate/ sodium bicarb	Oncology			1000	mL	x
METHOTREXate	Oncology		mg	100	mL	x
mitoxantrone	Oncology		mg	50	mL	x
natalizumab	Oncology	300	mg	100	mL	
nelarabine	Oncology	5	mg	1	mL	x
Other Drug	Oncology		Select on In-fuser		mL	
oxaliplatin	Oncology		mg	500	mL	x
PACLitaxel over 1 hr	Oncology		mg	250	mL	x
PACLitaxel over 3 hr	Oncology		mg	500	mL	x
PACLitaxel over 24 hr	Oncology		mg	500	mL	x
PACLitaxel prtn bd (abraxane)	Oncology	5	mg	1	mL	x
pegaspargase	Oncology		units	100	mL	x
pemetrexed	Oncology		mg	100	mL	x
pentostatin	Oncology		mg	50	mL	x
rasuricase	Oncology		mg	50	mL	x
rituximab	Oncology	1	mg	1	mL	x

Source: With permission from Fairview Health Services, Minneapolis, Minnesota.

Basic Enabled	Piggyback Enabled	Intermittent Enabled	Multistep Enabled	Delivery at End of Infusion	Default KVO Rate (mL/hr)	Enable Piggyback & Bolus From Secondary
x	x			KVO	10	
x	x			KVO	10	
x	x			KVO	10	
x	x			KVO	10	
x				KVO	10	
x	x			KVO	10	
x	x			KVO	10	
x	x			KVO	10	
x	x			KVO	10	
x	x			KVO	10	
x				KVO	10	
x	x			KVO	10	
x	x			KVO	10	
x				KVO	10	
x	x			KVO	10	
x	x			KVO	10	
x	x			KVO	10	
x	x			KVO	10	
x	x			KVO	10	
x	x			KVO	10	
x	x	x	x	KVO	1	x
x	x			KVO	10	x
x				KVO	10	x
x				KVO	10	
x	x			KVO	10	
x	x			KVO	10	
x				KVO	10	
x	x			KVO	10	
x	x			KVO	10	
x	x		x	KVO	10	

Source: With permission from Fairview Health Services, Minneapolis, Minnesota.

Table A-3. Drug Properties (cont'd)

Displayed Name	CCA Name	Med. Amt.	Med. Unit	Diluent Amt.	Diluent Unit	High Risk
streptozocin	Oncology		mg	100	mL	x
TEMSIRolimus	Oncology		mg	250	mL	x
teniposide	Oncology		mg	250	mL	x
teniposide	Oncology		mg	500	mL	x
teniposide	Oncology		mg	1000	mL	x
thiotepa	Oncology		mg	50	mL	x
thiotepa	Oncology		mg	100	mL	x
thiotepa	Oncology		mg	250	mL	x
topotecan	Oncology		mg	100	mL	x
TRASTuzumab over 30 min	Oncology		mg	250	mL	x
TRASTuzumab over 90 min	Oncology		mg	250	mL	x
vinBLAStine-infuse via gravity	Oncology		mg	25	mL	x
vinCRISTine	Oncology		mg	1000	mL	x
vinCRIStine infuse via gravity	Oncology		mg	25	mL	x
vinoRELBine infuse via gravity	Oncology		mg	25	mL	x
zoledronic acid	Oncology		mg	100	mL	
IV fluid	Outpt Infu				mL	
Premedication	Outpt Infu		mg		mL	
blood products	Outpt Infu				mL	x
potassium chloride	Outpt Infu	10	mEq	100	mL	
potassium chloride	Outpt Infu	20	mEq	50	mL	
magnesium replacement	Outpt Infu	1	grams	50	mL	
magnesium replacement	Outpt Infu		grams	100	mL	
antibiotic (except vancomycin)	Outpt Infu			50	mL	
antibiotic (except vancomycin)	Outpt Infu			100	mL	
antibiotic (except vancomycin)	Outpt Infu			150	mL	
antibiotic (except vancomycin)	Outpt Infu			250	mL	

Source: With permission from Fairview Health Services, Minneapolis, Minnesota.

Basic Enabled	Piggyback Enabled	Intermittent Enabled	Multistep Enabled	Delivery at End of Infusion	Default KVO Rate (mL/hr)	Enable Piggyback & Bolus From Secondary
x	x			KVO	10	
x	x			KVO	10	
x				KVO	10	
x				KVO	10	
x				KVO	10	
x	x			KVO	10	
x	x			KVO	10	
x				KVO	10	
x	x			KVO	10	
x				KVO	10	
x	x			KVO	10	
x				KVO	10	
x	x			KVO	10	
x				KVO	10	
x				KVO	10	
x	x			KVO	10	
x	x		x	KVO	10	x
x	x			KVO	10	
x				KVO	10	
x	x			KVO	10	
x	x			KVO	10	
x	x			KVO	10	
x	x			KVO	10	
x	x			KVO	10	
x	x			KVO	10	
x	x			KVO	10	
x	x			KVO	10	

Source: With permission from Fairview Health Services, Minneapolis, Minnesota.

Table A-3. Drug Properties (cont'd)

Displayed Name	CCA Name	Med. Amt.	Med. Unit	Diluent Amt.	Diluent Unit	High Risk
antibiotic (except vancomycin)	Outpt Infu			500	mL	
vancomycin	Outpt Infu		mg		mL	
abatacept	Outpt Infu		mg	100	mL	
calcium CHLORide	Outpt Infu		grams	100	mL	
calcium GLUConate	Outpt Infu	1	grams	100	mL	
ferric gluconate	Outpt Infu	125	mg	100	mL	
ferric gluconate	Outpt Infu	250	mg	250	mL	
immune globulin-sucrose out pat	Outpt Infu				mL	
immune globulin-sucrose free op	Outpt Infu				mL	
infliximab	Outpt Infu		mg	250	mL	
iron dextran test dose	Outpt Infu	25	mg	50	mL	
iron dextran	Outpt Infu		mg	500	mL	
iron sucrose (Venofer)	Outpt Infu	200	mg	100	mL	
iron sucrose (Venofer)	Outpt Infu	500	mg	250	mL	
mannitol injection 20%	Outpt Infu	50	grams	250	mL	
mannitol injection 20%	Outpt Infu	100	grams	500	mL	
mannitol injection 25%	Outpt Infu	12.5	grams	50	mL	
mannitol injection 25%	Outpt Infu		grams		mL	
methylprednisolone	Outpt Infu		mg	100	mL	
Other Drug	Outpt Infu		Select on In-fuser		mL	
pamidronate	Outpt Infu		mg	250	mL	
pamidronate	Outpt Infu		mg	500	mL	
pamidronate	Outpt Infu		mcg	1000	mL	
prolastin	Outpt Infu		mg		mL	
ranitidine intermittent	Outpt Infu	50	mg	50	mL	
thymoglobulin	Outpt Infu	50	mg	115	mL	
thymoglobulin	Outpt Infu	75	mg	173	mL	

Source: With permission from Fairview Health Services, Minneapolis, Minnesota.

Basic Enabled	Piggyback Enabled	Intermittent Enabled	Multistep Enabled	Delivery at End of Infusion	Default KVO Rate (mL/hr)	Enable Piggyback & Bolus From Secondary
x	x			KVO	10	
x	x			KVO	10	
x	x			KVO	10	
x	x			KVO	10	
x	x			KVO	10	
x	x			KVO	10	
x	x			KVO	10	
x				KVO	10	
x				KVO	10	
x	x			KVO	10	
x	x			KVO	10	
x	x			KVO	10	
x	x			KVO	10	
x	x			KVO	10	
x				KVO	10	
x				KVO	10	
x				KVO	10	
x				KVO	10	
x	x			KVO	10	
x	x	x	x	KVO	1	x
x				KVO	10	
x				KVO	10	
x				KVO	10	
x	x			KVO	10	
x	x	x	x	KVO	5	x
x	x			KVO	10	
x	x			KVO	10	

Source: With permission from Fairview Health Services, Minneapolis, Minnesota.

Table A-3. Drug Properties (cont'd)

Displayed Name	CCA Name	Med. Amt.	Med. Unit	Diluent Amt.	Diluent Unit	High Risk
thymoglobulin	Outpt Infu	100	mg	283	mL	
thymoglobulin-peripheral	Outpt Infu		mg	500	mL	
zoledronic acid	Outpt Infu		mg	100	mL	
IV fluid	adult bmt				mL	
calcium GLUConate	adult bmt	1	grams	100	mL	
cyclosporine	adult bmt		mg	100	mL	
cyclosporine	adult bmt		mg	150	mL	
cyclosporine	adult bmt		mg	250	mL	
cyclosporine drip BMT	adult bmt	250	mg	250	mL	
cyclosporine drip BMT	adult bmt	500	mg	250	mL	
filgrastim	adult bmt	15	mcg	1	mL	
foscarnet	adult bmt		mg		mL	
ganciclovir	adult bmt		mg	100	mL	x
lipids 20%	adult bmt	50	grams	250	mL	
lipids 20%	adult bmt	100	grams	500	mL	
magnesium replacement	adult bmt		grams		mL	
methylprednisolone	adult bmt		mg	100	mL	
phytonadione (vitamin K)	adult bmt		mg	50	mL	
potassium chloride	adult bmt	10	mEq	100	mL	
potassium chloride	adult bmt	20	mEq	50	mL	
potassium phosphate	adult bmt		mmol	500	mL	
potassium phosphate	adult bmt		mmol	250	mL	
sodium phosphate	adult bmt		mmol	250	mL	
sodium phosphate	adult bmt		mmol	500	mL	
TPN	adult bmt				mL	
3% sodium chloride	adult bmt				mL	x
AMIODarone	adult bmt	500	mg	500	mL	
AMIODarone	adult bmt	1500	mg	250	mL	
antibiotic (except vancomycin)	adult bmt			50	mL	
antibiotic (except vancomycin)	adult bmt			100	mL	

Source: With permission from Fairview Health Services, Minneapolis, Minnesota.

Basic Enabled	Piggyback Enabled	Intermittent Enabled	Multistep Enabled	Delivery at End of Infusion	Default KVO Rate (mL/hr)	Enable Piggyback & Bolus From Secondary
x	x			KVO	10	
x	x			KVO	10	
x	x			KVO	10	
x	x		x	KVO	10	x
x	x			KVO	10	
x	x			KVO	10	
x	x			KVO	10	
x	x			KVO	10	
x				Continue		
x				Continue		
x	x			KVO	10	
x				KVO	10	
x	x			KVO	10	
x				KVO	10	
x				KVO	10	
x	x			KVO	10	
x	x			KVO	10	
x	x			KVO	10	
x	x			KVO	10	
x	x			KVO	10	
x	x			KVO	10	
x	x			KVO	10	
x	x			KVO	10	
x			x	KVO	10	x
x				KVO	10	
x			x	Continue		
x			x	Continue		
x	x			KVO	10	
x	x			KVO	10	

Source: With permission from Fairview Health Services, Minneapolis, Minnesota.

Table A-3. Drug Properties (cont'd)

Displayed Name	CCA Name	Med. Amt.	Med. Unit	Diluent Amt.	Diluent Unit	High Risk
antibiotic (except vancomycin)	adult bmt			150	mL	
antibiotic (except vancomycin)	adult bmt			250	mL	
antibiotic (except vancomycin)	adult bmt			500	mL	
antithymocyte globulin horse	adult bmt		grams	250	mL	
antithymocyte globulin horse	adult bmt		grams	500	mL	
antithymocyte globulin horse	adult bmt		mg	150	mL	
bumetanide ICU	adult bmt	25	mg	100	mL	
chemo infusion	adult bmt				mL	x
calcium CHLORide	adult bmt		grams	100	mL	
chlorpromazine	adult bmt	25	mg	50	mL	
chlorpromazine	adult bmt	50	mg	100	mL	
cidofovir	adult bmt		mg	100	mL	
dantrolene	adult bmt		mg		mL	
desmopressin	adult bmt		mcg	50	mL	
diltiazem	adult bmt	125	mg	125	mL	
fentanyl	adult bmt	5	mg	100	mL	x
furosemide	adult bmt	100	mg	100	mL	
HEParin	adult bmt	25000	units	250	mL	x
HYDROmorphone	adult bmt		mg		mL	x
immune globulin-sucrose	adult bmt				mL	
immune globulin-sucrose free	adult bmt				mL	
ketamine	adult bmt		mg		mL	x
leucovorin	adult bmt	10	mg	1	mL	
levetiracetam	adult bmt			100	mL	
lorazepam	adult bmt	50	mg	50	mL	x
metoclopramide	adult bmt		mg	50	mL	
midazolam	adult bmt	50	mg	50	mL	x
morphine	adult bmt		mg		mL	x
mycophenolate 500 mg dose	adult bmt	500	mg		mL	

Source: With permission from Fairview Health Services, Minneapolis, Minnesota.

Basic Enabled	Piggyback Enabled	Intermittent Enabled	Multistep Enabled	Delivery at End of Infusion	Default KVO Rate (mL/hr)	Enable Piggyback & Bolus From Secondary
x	x			KVO	10	
x	x			KVO	10	
x	x			KVO	10	
x	x		x	KVO	10	
x	x		x	KVO	10	
x	x		x	KVO	10	
x				Continue		
x	x			KVO	10	
x	x			KVO	10	
x	x			KVO	10	
x	x			KVO	10	
x	x			KVO	10	
x	x			KVO	10	
x	x			KVO	10	
x				Continue		
x	x			Continue		
x				Continue		
x				Continue		
x	x			Continue		
x				KVO	10	
x				KVO	10	
x				Continue		
x	x		x	KVO	10	x
x	x			KVO	10	
x				Continue		
x	x		x	KVO	10	x
x				Continue		
x	x			Continue		
x				KVO	10	

Source: With permission from Fairview Health Services, Minneapolis, Minnesota.

Table A-3. Drug Properties (cont'd)

Displayed Name	CCA Name	Med. Amt.	Med. Unit	Diluent Amt.	Diluent Unit	High Risk
mycophenolate 1000 mg dose	adult bmt	1000	mg		mL	
mycophenolate 1500 mg dose	adult bmt	1500	mg		mL	
octreotide	adult bmt	1250	mcg	250	mL	
ondansetron drip	adult bmt	50	mg	50	mL	
Other Drug	adult bmt		Select on In-fuser		mL	
PANtoprazole	adult bmt	80	mg	100	mL	
premedication	adult bmt		mg	50	mL	
rituximab	adult bmt	1	mg	1	mL	x
sodium bicarbonate	adult bmt		mEq		mL	
tacrolimus	adult bmt	5	mg	250	mL	
thymoglobulin-BMT	adult bmt		mg	100	mL	
thymoglobulin-BMT	adult bmt		mg	150	mL	
thymoglobulin-BMT	adult bmt		mg	250	mL	
thymoglobulin-BMT	adult bmt		mg	500	mL	
vancomycin	adult bmt		mg		mL	
zoledronic acid	adult bmt		mg	100	mL	
Chemo over 30 min in ~50 mL	adult bmt			50	mL	x
Chemo over 30 min in ~100 mL	adult bmt			100	mL	x
Chemo over 30 min ~150 mL	adult bmt			150	mL	x
Chemo over 30 min in ~250 mL	adult bmt			250	mL	x
Chemo over 30 min in ~500 mL	adult bmt			500	mL	x
chemo over 1 hour ~100 mL	adult bmt			100	mL	x
chemo over 1 hour ~150 mL	adult bmt			150	mL	x
chemo over 1 hour ~250 mL	adult bmt			250	mL	x
Chemo over 1 hr in ~500 mL	adult bmt			500	mL	x
Chemo over 2 hr in ~100 mL	adult bmt			100	mL	x

Source: With permission from Fairview Health Services, Minneapolis, Minnesota.

Basic Enabled	Piggyback Enabled	Intermittent Enabled	Multistep Enabled	Delivery at End of Infusion	Default KVO Rate (mL/hr)	Enable Piggyback & Bolus From Secondary
x				KVO	10	
x				KVO	10	
x				Continue		
x	x			KVO	10	
x	x	x	x	KVO	1	x
x	x			Continue		
x	x			KVO	10	
x	x		x	KVO	10	
x	x			KVO	10	
x				Continue		
x	x			KVO	10	
x				KVO	10	
x				KVO	10	
x				KVO	10	
x	x			KVO	10	
x	x			KVO	10	
x	x			KVO	10	
x	x			KVO	10	
x	x			KVO	10	
x	x			KVO	10	
x	x			KVO	10	
x	x			KVO	10	
x	x			KVO	10	
x	x			KVO	10	
x	x			KVO	10	

Source: With permission from Fairview Health Services, Minneapolis, Minnesota.

Table A-3. Drug Properties (cont'd)

Displayed Name	CCA Name	Med. Amt.	Med. Unit	Diluent Amt.	Diluent Unit	High Risk
Chemo over 2 hr in ~ 150 mL	adult bmt			150	mL	x
Chemo over 2 hr in ~ 250 mL	adult bmt			250	mL	x
Chemo over 2 hr in ~ 500 mL	adult bmt			500	mL	x
Chemo over 3 hr in ~ 250 mL	adult bmt			250	mL	x
Chemo over 3 hr in ~ 500 mL	adult bmt			500	mL	x
Chemo over 24 hr in ~1000 mL	adult bmt			1000	mL	x
IV fluid	intermed				mL	
blood products	intermed				mL	x
antibiotic (except vancomycin)	intermed			50	mL	
antibiotic (except vancomycin)	intermed			100	mL	
antibiotic (except vancomycin)	intermed			150	mL	
antibiotic (except vancomycin)	intermed			250	mL	
antibiotic (except vancomycin)	intermed			500	mL	
AMIODarone	intermed	500	mg	500	mL	
AMIODarone	intermed	1500	mg	250	mL	
diltiazem	intermed	125	mg	125	mL	
HEParin	intermed	25000	units	250	mL	x
nitroGLYCERIN-IMC	intermed	50	mg	250	mL	x
nitroGLYCERIN-IMC	intermed	200	mg	250	mL	x
milrinone	intermed	20	mg	100	mL	x
furosemide	intermed	100	mg	100	mL	
DOBUTamine-IMC	intermed	500	mg	250	mL	x
DOBUTamine-IMC	intermed	1000	mg	250	mL	x
DOPamine-IMC	intermed	400	mg	250	mL	x
DOPamine-IMC	intermed	800	mg	250	mL	x
esmolol	intermed	2000	mg	100	mL	
potassium chloride	intermed	10	mEq	100	mL	
potassium chloride	intermed	20	mEq	50	mL	

Source: With permission from Fairview Health Services, Minneapolis, Minnesota.

Basic Enabled	Piggyback Enabled	Intermittent Enabled	Multistep Enabled	Delivery at End of Infusion	Default KVO Rate (mL/hr)	Enable Piggyback & Bolus From Secondary
x	x			KVO	10	
x	x			KVO	10	
x	x			KVO	10	
x	x			KVO	10	
x	x			KVO	10	
x	x			KVO	10	
x	x		x	KVO	10	x
x				KVO	10	
x	x			KVO	10	
x	x			KVO	10	
x	x			KVO	10	
x	x			KVO	10	
x	x			KVO	10	
x			x	Continue		
x			x	Continue		
x				Continue		
x				Continue		
x				Continue		
x				Continue		
x				Continue		
x				Continue		
x				Continue		
x				Continue		
x				Continue		
x				Continue		
x				Continue		
x	x			KVO	10	
x	x			KVO	10	

Source: With permission from Fairview Health Services, Minneapolis, Minnesota.

Table A-3. Drug Properties (cont'd)

Displayed Name	CCA Name	Med. Amt.	Med. Unit	Diluent Amt.	Diluent Unit	High Risk
TPN	intermed				mL	
lipids 20%	intermed	50	grams	250	mL	
lipids 20%	intermed	100	grams	500	mL	
magnesium replacement	intermed		grams		mL	
thymoglobulin	intermed	50	mg	115	mL	
thymoglobulin	intermed	75	mg	173	mL	
thymoglobulin	intermed	100	mg	283	mL	
thymoglobulin-peripheral	intermed		mg	500	mL	
immune globulin-sucrose	intermed				mL	
immune globulin-sucrose free	intermed				mL	
3% sodium chloride	intermed				mL	x
abciximab 80 kg or more	intermed	9	mg	250	mL	x
abciximab less than 80 kg	intermed	9	mg	250	mL	x
acetylcysteine-renal	intermed	600	mg	100	mL	
acetylcysteine-renal	intermed	1200	mg	100	mL	
alemtuzumab	intermed		mg	100	mL	x
alteplase PE	intermed	100	mg	100	mL	x
alteplase stroke	intermed		mg		mL	x
argatroban-cath lab	intermed	250	mg	250	mL	x
argatroban non-cath lab	intermed	250	mg	250	mL	x
basiliximab	intermed		mg	50	mL	
BEVACizumab over 30 min	intermed		mg	100	mL	x
BEVACizumab over 60 min	intermed		mg	100	mL	x
BEVACizumab over 90 min	intermed		mg	100	mL	x
bumetanide	intermed	25	mg	100	mL	
calcium CHLORide	intermed		grams	100	mL	
calcium GLUConate	intermed	1	grams	100	mL	
chlorpromazine	intermed	25	mg	50	mL	

Source: With permission from Fairview Health Services, Minneapolis, Minnesota.

Basic Enabled	Piggyback Enabled	Intermittent Enabled	Multistep Enabled	Delivery at End of Infusion	Default KVO Rate (mL/hr)	Enable Piggyback & Bolus From Secondary
x			x	KVO	10	x
x				KVO	10	
x				KVO	10	
x	x			KVO	10	
x	x			KVO	10	
x	x			KVO	10	
x	x			KVO	10	
x	x			KVO	10	
x				KVO	10	
x				KVO	10	
x				KVO	10	
x				Continue		
x				Continue		
x	x			KVO	10	
x	x			KVO	10	
x	x			KVO	10	
x				Continue		
x				Continue		
x				Continue		
x				Continue		
x				Continue		
x	x			KVO	10	
x	x			KVO	10	
x	x			KVO	10	x
x				Continue		x
x	x			KVO	10	
x	x			KVO	10	
x	x			KVO	10	

Source: With permission from Fairview Health Services, Minneapolis, Minnesota.

Table A-3. Drug Properties (cont'd)

Displayed Name	CCA Name	Med. Amt.	Med. Unit	Diluent Amt.	Diluent Unit	High Risk
chlorpromazine	intermed	50	mg	100	mL	
conivaptan	intermed	20	mg	250	mL	
cyclosporine drip-solid organ	intermed	250	mg	250	mL	
cyclosporine drip-solid organ	intermed	500	mg	250	mL	
daclizumab	intermed		mg	50	mL	
deferoxamine	intermed		mg	250	mL	
desmopressin	intermed		mcg	50	mL	
eptifibatide	intermed	200	mg	100	mL	x
ferric gluconate	intermed	125	mg	100	mL	
ferric gluconate	intermed	250	mg	250	mL	
foscarnet	intermed		mg		mL	
fosphenytoin	intermed		mg		mL	
ganciclovir	intermed		mg	100	mL	x
infliximab	intermed		mg	250	mL	
iron dextran	intermed		mg	500	mL	
iron dextran test dose	intermed	25	mg	50	mL	
iron sucrose (Venofer)	intermed	200	mg	100	mL	
iron sucrose (Venofer)	intermed	500	mg	250	mL	
isoproterenol-mcg/kg/min dosing	intermed	1	mg	50	mL	x
lepirudin	intermed	100	mg	250	mL	x
levetiracetam	intermed			100	mL	
mannitol injection 20%	intermed	50	grams	250	mL	
mannitol injection 20%	intermed	100	grams	500	mL	
mannitol injection 25%	intermed	12.5	grams	50	mL	
mannitol injection 25%	intermed		grams		mL	
methylprednisolone	intermed		mg	100	mL	
mycophenolate 500 mg dose	intermed	500	mg		mL	

Source: With permission from Fairview Health Services, Minneapolis, Minnesota.

Basic Enabled	Piggyback Enabled	Intermittent Enabled	Multistep Enabled	Delivery at End of Infusion	Default KVO Rate (mL/hr)	Enable Piggyback & Bolus From Secondary
x	x			KVO	10	
x				Continue		
x				Continue		
x				Continue		
x	x			KVO	10	
x	x			KVO	10	
x	x			KVO	10	
x				Continue		
x	x			KVO	10	
x	x			KVO	10	
x				KVO	10	
x				KVO	10	
x	x			KVO	10	
x	x			KVO	10	
x	x			KVO	10	
x	x			KVO	10	
x	x			KVO	10	
x	x			KVO	10	
x				Continue		
x				Continue		
x	x			KVO	10	
x				KVO	10	
x				KVO	10	
x				KVO	10	
x				KVO	10	
x	x			KVO	10	
x				KVO	10	

Source: With permission from Fairview Health Services, Minneapolis, Minnesota.

Table A-3. Drug Properties (cont'd)

Displayed Name	CCA Name	Med. Amt.	Med. Unit	Diluent Amt.	Diluent Unit	High Risk
mycophenolate 1000 mg dose	intermed	1000	mg		mL	
mycophenolate 1500 mg dose	intermed	1500	mg		mL	
naloxone	intermed	4	mg	100	mL	
octreotide	intermed	1250	mcg	250	mL	
ondansetron drip	intermed	50	mg	50	mL	
Other Drug	intermed		Select on In-fuser		mL	
PANtoprazole	intermed	80	mg	100	mL	
phytonadione (vita-min K)	intermed		mg	50	mL	
potassium phosphate	intermed		mmol	250	mL	
potassium phosphate	intermed		mmol	500	mL	
rituximab	intermed	1	mg	1	mL	x
sodium bicarbonate	intermed		mEq		mL	
sodium phosphate	intermed		mmol	250	mL	
sodium phosphate	intermed		mmol	500	mL	
tacrolimus	intermed	5	mg	250	mL	
tenecteplase	intermed	5	mg	500	mL	x
valproate	intermed		mg	100	mL	
vancomycin	intermed		mg		mL	

Source: With permission from Fairview Health Services, Minneapolis, Minnesota.

Basic Enabled	Piggyback Enabled	Intermittent Enabled	Multistep Enabled	Delivery at End of Infusion	Default KVO Rate (mL/hr)	Enable Piggyback & Bolus From Secondary
x				KVO	10	
x				KVO	10	
x				Continue		
x				Continue		
x	x			KVO	10	
x	x	x	x	KVO	1	x
x	x			Continue		
x	x			KVO	10	
x	x			KVO	10	
x	x			KVO	10	
x	x		x	KVO	10	
x	x			KVO	10	
x	x			KVO	10	
x	x			KVO	10	
x				Continue		
x	x			KVO	10	
x	x			KVO	10	
x	x			KVO	10	

Source: With permission from Fairview Health Services, Minneapolis, Minnesota.

Glossary

510(k) clearance—Section 510(k) of the Food, Drug, and Cosmetic Act requires device manufacturers to notify the FDA of their intent to market a medical device at least 90 days in advance. High-risk devices are designated at Class III, and require 510(k) clearance prior to marketing.

Adult patient—a patient 17 years old and weighing at least 45 kilograms.

Alert fatigue—a tendency to ignore or minimize the potential negative impact of a technology alert, when presented with multiple alerts with varying degrees of importance.

Bar code medication administration (BCMA)—technology that involves placing a unique identifier that is machine readable by an optical scanner on each medication.

Biomedical services—department within the health system concerned with storing and maintaining biomedical equipment and technology.

Bolus dose—a medication dose meant to be delivered over a very short period of time.

Commercial product—sterile drug that has been evaluated by the Food and Drug Administration (FDA) for safety and efficacy.

Compounding—preparation, mixing, assembling, packaging, and labeling of a drug or device.

Clinical care area (see also Drug library subset)—an area of the health system representing a certain group of patients who have similar patient care needs. For purposes of the infusion pump, a clinical care area is part of the pump programming that allows medications needed in the particular area to be separated into one particular list for one particular area. One example of a clinical care area is "Intensive Care Unit."

Clinician compliance—the extent to which caregivers use the pump as was intended; programming the pump using the safety software.

Critical criteria—criteria chosen by a selection team. These criteria, when present, are thought to bring a higher value to the object being evaluated.

Dose error reduction system (DERS)—a term used to describe software built into intelligent infusion devices that is designed to catch dosing or administration errors. In this case, it represents the programming of minimum and maximum dose limits in an infusion pump, and the alerts presented to the clinician when programmed doses are exceeded.

Dose rate units—units used to express the rate of infusion of a drug.

Dose variables—drug selection, initial loading dose, PCA dose, lockout interval, infusion rate, dose limits.

Drug library—a comprehensive list of medications and fluids that are to be delivered using the infusion pump. This library includes any dose, volume, or rate limitations that are programmed into the software.

Drug dataset—used interchangeably with drug library (see above).

Drug library push—the act of updating pumps using wireless technology. The new drug library is "pushed" from the software housing the library out to the individual pumps.

Drug library subset—a subset of the larger drug library that includes all drugs needed for a specific patient population or area. Other names that pump vendors use for these subsets are personalities, profiles, and clinical care areas.

DL—drug library.

EMR—electronic medical record.

Entity—single factor within the health system (individual hospital, clinic, or infusion center).

Failure modes and effects analysis (FMEA)—a process where potential failures of a device or system are uncovered.

"Hard" dose limit—a dose limit programmed into a pump; the pump cannot be programmed outside a "hard" limit. The user must use a dose within the hard limits.

High "hard" dose limit—a high dose limit programmed into a pump; the pump cannot be programmed higher than a high "hard" limit. The user must use a dose lower than this limit.

High "soft" dose limit—a high dose limit programmed into a pump; the pump will alert the user that the dose is unusually high, however, the user can still proceed with programming this dose.

Human factors techniques—the study of human interactions with devices.

Infusion pump—a device that uses pressure to deliver specific volumes of fluid; used for fluid, blood and medication administration.

IS—information services.

Large volume pump—an infusion device used to deliver medications for which a very small volume or rate of infusion is not necessary.

Line labels—the practice of labeling infusion tubing in order to identify which medication is infusing in the tubing. For purposes of the smart pumps, the pump will display the drug name on the pump itself, perhaps obviating the need to label tubing lines.

Low "hard" dose limit—a low dose limit programmed into a pump; the pump cannot be programmed lower than a low "hard" limit. The user must use a dose higher than this limit.

Low "soft" dose limit—a low dose limit programmed into a pump; the pump will alert the user that the dose is unusually low, however, the user can still proceed with programming this dose.

MAUDE—the Manufacturer and User Facility Device Experience is an online database maintained by the FDA. MAUDE data represents voluntary reports of adverse events involving medical devices.

Minimum effective analgesic concentration (MEAC)—the lowest steady-state serum concentration of an analgesic medication at which pain is relieved.

Mode of administration (delivery mode)—PCA dose only, continuous infusion only, PCA dose plus continuous infusion.

National drug code (NDC)—medication identity for commercial products, which includes the drug company labeling, drug name, dose, and package size.

Neonatal patient—a patient less than 1 month old.

Nesting—grouping varying drug concentrations under a single drug name. This avoids having both concentrations show up on the main screen, thereby avoiding excessive scrolling.

Overrides—the action of continuing to program the pump at the bedside with entered doses, concentrations, or rates despite receiving high or low dose alerts.

Password protection—some pumps offer the added feature of requiring a password code to be input in order to gain access to a medication library, if the library is thought to include particularly high-risk medications, concentrations, or dose limits.

PCA basal rate (continuous infusion, background infusion)—an analgesic medication administered at a constant rate (mg/hr or mcg/hr).

Patient controlled analgesia (PCA)—a conceptual framework for administration of analgesics to provide immediate delivery of the medication upon patient demand. PCA is not restricted to a single class of analgesics, routes, or modes of administration (for example, IV–PCA, epidural–PCEA).

PCA demand dose (PCA dose, incremental dose)—quantity of an analgesic medication administered by the patient upon activation of the dose button linked to the PCA pump.

PCA dose limit—total amount of an analgesic medication that can be given in any 1-hour or 4-hour period.

PCA loading dose (bolus dose)—clinician (nurse or physician) activated dose administered through the PCA pump for initial titration to the MEAC.

PCA time interval (lockout)—minimum allowable period between patient-activated PCA doses.

Pediatric patient—a patient older than 1 month, but less than 17 years and weighing less than 45 kilograms.

Piggyback dose—a medication dose meant to be delivered over a relatively short period of time; this medication is meant to be infused through a pump via a connection between the pump tubing and the medication tubing.

Pump edits—the action of modifying pump programming at the bedside in response to a high or low dose alert.

Request for proposal—a request for proposal (referred to as RFP) is an invitation for suppliers, often through a bidding process, to submit a proposal for a specific commodity or service.

Return on investment (ROI)—a performance measure used to evaluate the efficiency of an investment.

Safety software—see definition for DERS, above.

Scrolling—reading through drug names on the pump in order to find the desired drug name. If a drug list is fairly long, excessive scrolling can be inefficient.

Smart infusion pumps—a new generation of infusion pumps that incorporates dose limiting software into the pump hardware; this software is designed to prevent infusion-related programming errors. The Joint Commission, in the 2006 National Patient Safety Goals, defined a smart pump as a "Parenteral infusion pump equipped with IV medication error-prevention software that alerts operators or interrupts the infusion process when a pump setting is programmed outside of pre-configured limits. Smart pumps are designed to recognize prescription errors, dose misinterpretations, and keypad programming errors."

"Soft" dose limit—a dose limit programmed into a pump; the pump will alert the user that the dose is unusual, however, the user can still proceed with programming this dose.

Sterile services—department within the health system concerned with cleaning and sterilizing supplies.

Super-users—individuals involved in the selection and implementation of smart pumps who feel familiar enough with the processes to educate others. Super-users may be relied upon to mentor other users not as familiar with the technology. Super-users may also conduct formal training sessions.

Supply chain—department within the health system concerned with obtaining products and supplies from vendors.

Syringe pump—an infusion device used to deliver medications that require a very small volume or rate of infusion.

System—all entities within the health system.

Tall-man lettering—a means of depicting drug names so that similar looking names can be differentiated. The part of the name that differentiates the two drugs is labeled with capital letters (for example, DOPamine, DOBUTamine).

Usability testing—a test to determine how well a device functions in a real-life scenarios.

Value analysis—a systematic, objective means to measure the value of an object (usability divided by cost) in comparison to other like objects.

Weighted decision matrix—the process of assigning numerical values to object attributes; the higher the number, the more important the attribute. If an object performs exceptionally well in an attribute with a high matrix value, it is thought to provide more value overall.

Index